Leadership for
GREAT
CUSTOMER
SERVICE

Leadership for GREAT CUSTOMER SERVICE

Satisfied Employees, Satisfied Patients

SECOND EDITION

THOM A. MAYER & ROBERT J. CATES

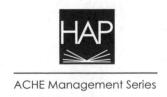

ACHE Management Series

Your board, staff, or clients may also benefit from this book's insight. For more information on quantity discounts, contact the Health Administration Press Marketing Manager at (312) 424-9470.

18   17   16   15   5   4   3   2

Library of Congress Cataloging-in-Publication Data

Mayer, Thom A.
  Leadership for great customer service : satisfied employees, satisfied patients / Thom A. Mayer and Robert J. Cates. — Second edition.
     pages cm
  ISBN 978-1-56793-642-1 (alk. paper)
  1. Patient satisfaction. 2. Medical personnel and patient. 3. Medical care—Quality control. I. Cates, Robert J. II. Title.
  R727.3.M385 2014
  610.69'6—dc23
                       2014009162

The paper used in this publication meets the minimum requirements of American National Standard for Information Sciences—Permanence of Paper for Printed Library Materials, ANSI Z39.48-1984.∞™

Acquisitions editor: Tulie O'Connor; Project manager: Joyce Dunne; Cover designer: Renee Duenow; Layout: PerfecType

Found an error or a typo? We want to know! Please e-mail it to hapbooks@ache.org, and put "Book Error" in the subject line.

For photocopying and copyright information, please contact Copyright Clearance Center at www.copyright. com or at (978) 750-8400.

Health Administration Press
A division of the Foundation of the American
   College of Healthcare Executives
One North Franklin Street, Suite 1700
Chicago, IL 60606-3529
(312) 424-2800

To my beautiful, brilliant, and always inspiring wife, Maureen—you have been and will always be the most amazing person in the world;

To our sons, Greg, Kevin, and Josh—your humor, kindness, and courage are testaments to the future we all aspire toward;

To Josh's wife, Valerie, and their wonderful daughters, Eve and Audra, who are delightful, gracious, and generous;

To the memory of my parents, affectionately known as Grandpa Jim and Grandma Bette, your wisdom, I hope and pray, is somehow reflected, however imperfectly, in these pages;

To the memory of Maureen's father, John B. Henry, MD, who was a scientist, physician, and man of substance and style; and

To Maureen's elegant mother, Georgette, who gave me the greatest gift in my life—her daughter.

Thom Mayer, MD

To my wife, Kim; my children, Beth, Rob, Jill, and Sarah; and my sister, Debbie, in appreciation of your love and support.

Robert J. Cates, MD

In memory of our
trusted colleagues and dear friends
Martin Gottlieb
Joan Kyes, RN
Stephen Dresnick, MD, FACEP

Contents

Part II: Survival Skills for Achieving Great Customer Service

Foreword to the Second Edition

In 2004, when the first edition of *Leadership for Great Customer Service* was published, the notion that treating patients as human beings was good for business was still new. In fact, there was fierce resistance to paying attention to patient satisfaction, which was often dismissed as whimpering about dirty rooms and rude, incommunicative nurses. Healthcare meant the important business of clinical quality, end of story.

In 2014, some clinicians remain resistant, but the tectonic plates underneath this industry are shifting, creating an entirely new landscape. The regulatory environment is now suffused with terms such as *value-based purchasing, HCAHPS*, and *the patient experience of care*. The advent of accountable care organizations, medical homes, and bundled payment networks—population health management—requires providers to keep patients loyal and in network to have any chance of success.

The economic terrain is also seismically unstable as retail clinics, hospitals at home, and mobile health solutions emerge as competition. Employers are pushing workers into high-deductible health plans, and the new marketplace plans under reform also take more from people's pocketbooks. Consumers now have a world of choices in accessing care and are far more cost-conscious than in the past. They make decisions based in large measure on how they feel about their prior experiences. That means hospitals, health systems, medical practices, and ambulatory care providers had better get with the program of good customer service as a core strategy for survival. It's a jungle out there, so it's time to treat patients as if they are your lifeblood. Trust me, they are.

In this concise, penetrating, and entertaining update of their earlier work, Doctors Thom Mayer and Robert Cates show how patients have come to expect both clinical quality and service quality, which are inextricably linked. Numerous studies now underscore this connection: Outcomes are affected when patients feel mistreated, no matter how appropriate or "successful" the clinical treatment. Gaining buy-in from hospital employees for any new customer service initiative is critical, the authors show. They ought to know, having conducted hundreds of customer service training sessions in hospitals. They use the analogy of "renters versus owners" such that owners are fully engaged in the organization's success and view their roles as responsibilities, whereas renters just show up and do the minimum to get paid, viewing their roles as jobs. Mayer and Cates make it clear that selecting people with positive attitudes and giving them the right training are essential strategies.

Full disclosure: I have been writing about the importance of good customer service in healthcare and other industries for decades. Mayer and Cates demonstrate how the CEO needs to explain why customer service is important to frontline caregivers as well as how to get service right. Without giving away too much, they show how treating patients with empathy and caring makes everyone's job easier, not harder.

A good friend of mine, Paul Spiegelman, JD, along with his coauthor, Britt Berrett, PhD, FACHE, recently published a book entitled *Patients Come Second* (An Inc. Original, 2013). In their introduction they acknowledge that their title is controversial, but it reflects the importance of focusing first on healthcare workers, engaging them openly and honestly about the "why" of customer service. Some of them may never "get it," but most should feel energized when they understand the link to making their jobs more fulfilling and improving patient outcomes.

If you asked people in this industry who their boss is, most would say the chief medical officer or the head nurse or the CEO. We hear much talk about patient-centered care, and I have no doubt that, for some people and organizations, it really is their mission. But viewing the patient as the boss takes patient-centered care to a different level. Patients and families walk into the lobby of a hospital looking anxious and uncertain of where to go. When they ask a passing hospital employee where outpatient surgery or radiology is, the employee often wordlessly points down a long corridor filled with signs and doorways. When the patient is your boss, you escort her down the hallway, introduce her to the person she needs to see, and thank her for the opportunity to serve her needs. Only then do you return to your previous task.

Sharon Brooks did that for me. I was at Rush University Medical Center in Chicago, having blood drawn for my upcoming hip replacement surgery, and I have to admit I was a little nervous. Usually when I go through the bureaucratic process of registration, I wind up offended. Often there is little eye contact and no reassuring smile or other personal touch at a time when you could use it. But at Rush, not only did Sharon smile but she took care of me. She gave me strips of stickers that say "Smiles are Contagious—Catch One!" She was so full of energy, enthusiasm, and goodwill that I couldn't help noticing. After she got all the information she needed, she brought out a machine that blew soap bubbles. Everyone in the admitting area was smiling, even those who were clearly there for something far more serious than I was. Sharon has probably done more for the image of the hospital than any expensive advertising campaign could do.

Leadership for Great Customer Service is about more than just how to make a good first impression. It is about how to create a culture where everyone, from the housekeeper to the CEO, views the mission of the organization to be the delivery of the highest-quality care—for both body and spirit. Healthcare providers that really understand this message will be the ones left standing when the earth stops shaking.

Chuck Lauer, HFACHE
Winnetka, Illinois

Foreword to the First Edition

In the madness of the modern world of healthcare, write Doctors Thom Mayer and Robert Cates in *Leadership for Great Customer Service*, technical excellence is a necessary but insufficient condition for institutional survival. The missing link, they argue persuasively (and based on an impressive body of research and "clinical practice" with service initiatives), is a strategic and cultural commitment to excellent customer service.

I honestly can't remember when I've seen so much of so much importance crammed into a short book. The authors do an excellent job of making the case for customer service excellence in acute care institutions. They go on to provide assistance in making the case with staffs. Then they lay out, with surpassing clarity, the process for embedding a service excellence culture in a medical institution. Finally, they devote the last third of the book to the details of program implementation, down to the important role of body language in patient–staff interactions. They do all of this in a little over a hundred pages, which are almost breezy (while serious) and jargon free, though written specifically for the healthcare professional. All in all, this is a masterful effort, and one that is long overdue.

Without (I hope) giving away the punch line, let me share in summary form my highlights tape:

- Customer service initiatives don't work unless they make the job easier for staff. Hint: They can!
- It takes a revolution. "All this" is more than a program, it's a *way of life*, a cultural about-face, lived strategically and in the grubby moment-to-moment details.
- There are A-team players and B-team players. B-team players are probably in the wrong job, and one at any level can destroy an entire shift. Deal with it: Work assiduously on improvement, and dump those who in the end don't/can't/won't get it.
- There is an enormous difference between a patient and a customer. Customers are vertical. Patients are horizontal. The majority of throughput is customers, and customers require a very different approach than patients. (The discussion of working with staff on identifying biases and clarifying definitions is worth the price of admission alone.)
- The service diagnosis is as important as the clinical diagnosis. And the approach to the two diagnoses is very different.

- Even in the lofty atmosphere of acute care medicine, one can, on occasion, turn an angry customer-patient into a friend and fan with a $25 gift certificate to Outback Steakhouse.
- Service excellence ultimately depends on the management of *moments of truth*, a collection of usually small incidents involving staff–patient interaction. These can be clearly identified, and responses can be meticulously scripted.
- Never cross your arms while talking to a patient-customer.

And so on.

In fact, a lot of this is right out of the Disney–Nordstrom playbook (though one of the authors had a single, nasty experience with Nordstrom—and never went back). Mayer and Cates acknowledge their debt to such exemplary institutions but point out that healthcare professionals have great difficulty (understatement, in my experience) analogizing from the pixie-dust world of Disney to the life-and-death world of emergency services. Make no mistake, while the lessons here are indeed universal, they come from healthcare research and program implementation, use healthcare cases, are couched in healthcare language, and deal with healthcare "objections."

Leadership for Great Customer Service is laserlike in its aim. It is not a screed on lousy service. It is not an Rx for healthcare in general. It is a terse, complete, focused, readable, at times amusing guide to addressing perhaps the number one opportunity for any acute care institution to win customer affection while making the working environment and staff's life more attractive simultaneously. Not a bad deal!

Tom Peters
Lenox, Massachusetts

Acknowledgments

It is impossible to overstate how gratified we have been with the overwhelmingly positive reception of the first edition of *Leadership for Great Customer Service: Satisfied Patients, Satisfied Employees*. While the positive reviews and substantial sales have been very much appreciated, by far the most important development for us has been the countless letters, phone calls, and e-mails we have received from dedicated healthcare providers and leaders across the United States—indeed, the world—telling us how helpful the book and its message have been. Our primary debt of gratitude is to those people and the patients they serve with great care on a daily basis. Without them, we would have had no reason to write a book in the first place. Our friend and colleague, Harry Rhoads Jr., cofounder of the Washington Speakers Bureau, has told us repeatedly, "The only reason to ever give a speech is to help someone." It is equally true of writing a book, and our deepest hope is that something in this text will make the difficult job of caring for patients easier for those who read it and better for the patients for whom they care.

No book is ever the sole product of the authors. Instead, any book reflects the complex interactions of the many, many people with whom the authors have worked to produce the thoughts reflected in their writing. In our case, this set of interactions is expanded exponentially by the tens of thousands of participants in our Survival Skills courses with whom we have connected over a 20-year period to refine these concepts.

We have always said that we are merely communicating the collective wisdom of the healthcare providers with whom we have worked. Our first debt, then, is to those who attended our courses. Our colleagues at BestPractices, Inc., and Inova Fairfax Hospital have been supportive of our efforts and exemplify daily the best in healthcare customer service. The emergency department nurses with whom we have worked at Inova Health System, Sentara Northern Virginia Medical Center, Susquehanna Health, Waterbury Hospital, St. Mary Medical Center, and many other facilities have enriched our lives beyond measure and have contributed to many of the concepts and strategies reflected in this book.

The members of the Physician Leadership Team at BestPractices are as fine a team of healthcare leaders as any in the nation, and their thoughts have contributed to the development of the Survival Skills concepts. They include Doctors Glenn Druckenbrod, John Howell, Rick Place, Kaidi Fullerton, John Maguire, Alan Lo, Alice Gouvenayre, David Postelnek, Mary Ann McLaurin, Hannah Grausz, Dan Hanfling, Scott Weir, Ron Thomas, Peter Jacoby, Praveen Kache, and Dan Avstreigh.

A special thanks to our business partner and colleague, Dr. Kirk Jensen, whose work on flow and its importance to the patient experience is immeasurable. He is a friend, colleague, and mentor to whom we are deeply grateful. To be able to work with him on a daily basis is a great honor and privilege.

We have had the good fortune to work with some of the finest healthcare administrators in the country, all of whom have been supportive of our commitment to customer service, including J. Knox Singleton; Mark Stauder; Patrick Christiansen; Toni Ardabell; Steven E. Brown, FACHE; Mary Jane Mastorovich; Edward R. Eroe, FACHE; Charles J. Barnett, FACHE; William Flanagan Jr.; William M. Moss, LFACHE; Joan Miles; Tom Corder; Megan Perry; David Schwartz, MD; Chad W. Wable, FACHE; John Moynihan, MD, FACS; and Richard J. Stull II. Without their support, the team nature of Survival Skills training could not have developed in the compelling fashion it has.

Linda Cooper is the finest administrative assistant in the world, and she is emblematic of the positive message of customer service. She was patient and painstakingly attentive to every detail in the creation and submission of this manuscript. Simply stated, the book could not have been completed without her excellent work. Her efforts are also appreciated during the scheduling of the Survival Skills training sessions, where her service talents exceed ours by a wide margin.

For more than 30 years, Kaye Wear was our practice manager and, in many ways, the soul of our physician group. Her kindness and generosity are exceeded only by her wisdom.

Many thanks to Tom Peters, both for contributing his generous and thoughtful foreword to the first edition of this book and for his friendship and mentoring over the years. To have the guidance of such an internationally recognized thought leader is fortune beyond belief.

Since the merger of BestPractices with EmCare and Envision Healthcare, it has been a privilege to work with Todd Zimmerman; Jay Taylor; Bill Sanger; and Drs. Dighton Packard, Russ Harris, Terry Meadows, and Angel Iscovich. Dr. Leonard Riggs, EmCare's founder, always embodied a deep commitment to customer service throughout the organization, and we are proud to be a part of that tradition.

For their patience with 20 years of hard work, long hours, and travel to every corner of the country, I (Thom) thank my wonderful wife, Maureen, and our sons, Josh, Kevin, and Gregory. Without their understanding and forbearance, neither the Survival Skills concept nor this book would have happened.

For her unwavering support, abundant wisdom, and uncommon common sense, I (Bob) thank my wife, Kim, and my four children, Beth, Rob, Jill, and Sarah, who continually teach me.

Janet Davis and Tulio O'Connor at Health Administration Press are experienced, insightful, and highly professional acquisitions editors who improved both the content and the presentation of this work. No authors could ask for better assistance, insight, and humor in the editorial process. They have made countless suggestions that have sharpened the manuscript's message, as well as making a difficult process fun and rewarding.

Joyce Dunne, our senior editor at Health Administration Press, transformed our manuscript into a far more polished and understandable final product, and we are deeply grateful for her wisdom, professionalism, and understanding.

To our friend and colleague Dr. Irwin Press goes our deepest respect and admiration for the many conversations we have had over the years regarding patient satisfaction and how best to attain it. Chuck Lauer, HFACHE, is arguably the most respected name in healthcare journalism, and we appreciate his insights and his friendship. Chuck Stokes, FACHE, is as fine a healthcare leader as there is, and he has mentored countless others, including us.

We have enjoyed our interaction and close working relationship with Quint Studer for more than 20 years. His insights have been of immeasurable help to us and to thousands of others.

Dr. Robert Strauss is not only a friend and colleague who has enriched our insights and our lives but also a national treasure in his wisdom regarding customer service.

Joan Kyes, RN, was an essential part of the birth of the Survival Skills concept. Her insights on stress, change management, and human behavior are critical to the development of this book and the course on which it was based. Her friendship, guidance, and humor enriched not only this book but our lives as well. Her untimely passing has left a void in our lives that is simply unfillable.

If we have neglected to mention the many others who have contributed to our lives and our thinking about customer service, it is only because of space limitations and does not reflect the depth of our gratitude and appreciation.

Part I

FRAMING THE CUSTOMER SERVICE MANDATE

CHAPTER 1

Getting Started: Why Worry About Customer Service in Healthcare?

One of the most intriguing and troubling questions facing healthcare leaders is, *How do I create a meaningful and lasting culture of customer service in my institution?* Improving customer service and patient satisfaction is a critical issue in administrative offices and hospital boardrooms across the United States.

THE IMPORTANCE OF HEALTHCARE CUSTOMER SERVICE: AN INTRODUCTION

More than a hundred books have been written on the application of customer service to healthcare. Many, if not most, healthcare leaders' core goals and objectives for the hospital (and their bonuses) are tied at least in part to attaining improved service excellence ratings. The problem, of course, is that while there is plenty of legitimate and genuine concern in the executive suite, too little practical guidance is provided in the patient care areas, where clinical care and customer service are offered. In other words, the *intention* is almost universally good, but the *execution* is often lacking. Despite posting eloquent mission statements, paying substantial fees to consultants, developing training materials and building sophisticated websites, and delivering appropriately passionate statements at management team meetings to exhort the troops, for many healthcare institutions, when it comes to customer service, the words and the music don't match.

Consider this example: Your organization has a first-rate service excellence road map, fully supported by fiercely passionate members of your leadership team. You've done the "tent revival" rollout, brought in the best motivational speakers, put up all the right posters and slogans in all the right places, and built accountability into the compensation plans of the entire management team. There's only one problem—the needle isn't moving up on the customer service gauge. As a matter of fact, it shows a disturbing downward trend.

Unfortunately, this is an increasingly common scenario, and one that has a single root cause: For many healthcare providers, the *why* of service excellence is much less clear than the *how*. But without a clear sense of why things are being done, the specific methods constituting the "how" get lost in the shuffle.

Nietzsche, in *Beyond Good and Evil*, made the point concisely:

He who has a strong enough "Why" can bear almost any "How."

> Between the idea
> And the reality
> Between the motion
> And the act
> Falls the shadow.
> —T. S. Eliot, *The Hollow Men*

Why is there such a long shadow between the *idea* of service excellence and the *reality* required to bring it to fruition? Why is there such a gap between the proclaimed commitment to and the actual delivery of customer service in healthcare institutions? Noted scholar of organizational behavior Chris Argyris (1993) comments, "For many institutions, the fundamental problem is the dissonance between the espoused strategy and the enacted strategy."

Part of the reason for the dissonance between the carefully espoused strategies of customer service and the enacted strategies seen in the patient care areas is that the staff members, charged with providing the service and enacting the strategy, can clearly understand why it is important to the CEO but not why it is important to *them*. As the old story goes (adapted from Belasco and Stayer 1993),

The CEO of a large regional healthcare system took one of her key managers to the top of a hill overlooking the city. Pointing down at a ridge just below them, she said, "Imagine a beautiful house sitting atop that ridge, overlooking the city. Can you see it?" "Oh yes, I can see it," said the manager. She continued, "Imagine there is a swimming pool just behind the house. Can you see it in your mind?" "Yes, yes I can!" said the manager, getting more excited. "Imagine there is something off to the right of the house—it's a tennis court! Can you see it?" "Yes," said the manager, "I can see it!" The CEO continued, "If this customer service initiative is successful and we continue to increase our market share, someday all of that will be . . . mine."

This concept can be illustrated in another way, through the lens of "owners" versus "renters." Owners are fully engaged in the organization's success; deeply passionate about its mission, vision, and values; and grateful for the opportunity to serve patients and their families. Renters? Well, they just show up, expecting a paycheck (and eventually a promotion) for their "time served." In a study of companies that were able to sustain their success, Jim Collins (2010) put it this way:

> One notable difference between wrong people and right people is that the former see themselves as having "jobs," while the latter see themselves as having "responsibilities."

Throughout this book, we show you how to make the distinction between owners and renters and those with jobs versus responsibilities clear and actionable in your organization. It starts with acknowledging a simple, yet often overlooked, consideration: Patients have come to expect *both* clinical quality and service quality, not one or the other. Thus, clinical excellence and service excellence cannot be separated—they are inextricably linked. When it comes to service and clinical quality, the framework through which it is achieved must always be based on "both/and," never "either/or" (discussed in detail later in the book).

This book is written for healthcare leaders operating at every level of the organization, with the understanding that transformation to a culture of service excellence requires not just the *intention* of the leadership but also the constant *attention* of doctors, nurses, radiology technicians, laboratory technicians, registrars, housekeepers, and so on across the organization. For this reason, our intent is to give *you* direction on how to give *them* direction to accomplish high-level customer service.

Toward this end, we present an approach that leaders can use to address those staff who provide service. We give you plenty of clinical examples of what you need to do to not only demonstrate your commitment to service excellence but also show clinicians *how* to apply highly successful strategies. Our greatest hope is that you will finish this book, hand it to your leadership team, and say, "Put this into action!" If you do, you *will* transform your organization.

Many in healthcare feel they are "at the ramparts," evoking images of a besieged, embattled industry facing declining revenues, increasing demands, an aging population, healthcare personnel shortages, emergency department crowding and diversion, and the reality that key providers of service—physicians—are typically neither employed nor controlled by the healthcare system. Into the midst of such difficulties comes the demand for improved customer service and patient satisfaction. Add to this the challenges of moving from volume-based to value-based purchasing and of adopting, adapting, and implementing different structures to comply with the Affordable Care Act, and healthcare providers may legitimately ask themselves, Is this *really* the time to be focusing on customer service in healthcare?

This honest and straightforward question deserves a frank and direct answer— "Yes!"—but for a reason that is not necessarily obvious, since it focuses more on the healthcare professional than on the patient. Having taught the customer service training course (Patient Care Survival Skills™) on which this book is based to more than 200,000 healthcare professionals for 20 years at more than 2,000 healthcare institutions, we have found that the most significant challenge to creating a culture of customer service is providing healthcare leaders and the healthcare team a clear and practical understanding of why customer service and patient satisfaction should be important to them. (We know it's important to you—indeed, your job may depend on it.) To do so, we pose to them—and you—a simple exercise. First, take a moment to consider the following statement.

The number one reason to get customer service right in healthcare is _____.

If you are like the many healthcare providers to whom we have given this exercise, your answers generally fall under the following classifications:

- It's better for the patient.
- It's better for the family.
- It's better for quality care.
- It's better for the medical staff.

- It's better for market share.
- It's better for risk management.
- It's better for reimbursement.
- It's better for patient safety.

The most commonly heard answer is that excellent customer service is good for the patient or the family. We also typically hear that it is good for risk reduction—those providers who are good at service are sued for malpractice at much lower rates than those who do not excel in that area, a fact that has been repeatedly demonstrated by Dr. Gerald Hickson (2009) and his colleagues at Vanderbilt University Medical Center.

All of these are great reasons to get customer service right in healthcare, but who primarily benefits—the individuals providing the services, or those who lead and manage the organization? As suggested by the first point in the right-hand column of the above list, market share improves when customer service improves. Sounds great—but what if I'm a nurse in a busy, overcrowded emergency department? The reward for good customer service is . . . *more patients*? That doesn't sound like a reward to us, nor will it to the nurses.

GETTING THE "WHY" RIGHT BEFORE ATTEMPTING THE "HOW"

Health leaders have spent an enormous amount of time, energy, and effort emphasizing and training for the "how to do it" questions of customer service while neglecting the "why do it in the first place" motivation, which is where we must always start.

Any customer service initiative that answers, "Why are we doing this?" with, "Because the boss says so" or "It's good for market share" is doomed to failure. In fact, such a response is precisely why most customer service initiatives in healthcare either fail or are not sustainable. The paradox is that, while all of the above responses are certainly true—and in themselves excellent reasons for getting customer service right—they miss the fundamental point:

The number one reason to get customer service right in healthcare is that
it makes the job easier.

Effecting change in service behaviors in the healthcare environment is nearly impossible unless the people providing the care understand this truth. *Anything* that is described as customer service should make the job easier. Make no mistake—providing clinical care at the bedside is a difficult job that seems to get more difficult each day. If we now say, "Oh, and by the way, get your customer service scores up, too," we should never be surprised if our staff members are not only not on board but ready to revolt. For that reason, there are two simple litmus tests for whether to launch a customer service initiative and the programs comprising them:

It's called customer service, but

1. *does* it make the job easier? If so,
2. *how* does it make the job easier?

If any initiative that is described as customer service fails either test, the staff providing the care know that it is not a true customer service–oriented effort. Further, they understand that things that come labeled as customer service but that do not make their jobs easier actually create *more work* for them. The translation of this knowledge to the work of healthcare delivery is one of the reasons so many service excellence initiatives in healthcare either fall short of their goals or produce temporary results rather than lasting cultural changes.

Rather than a vague management plan, service excellence is an *evidence-based discipline* designed to make the difficult job of patient care easier. Each of the ten elements of the A-Team Tool Kit, which are discussed in detail in Part III of the book, are not "rah-rah" cheerleading concepts or exhortations to raise scores. They are evidence-based solutions that were born of and proven over time to effect change by *making the job easier.*

How do we (1) communicate this solution-based approach to service excellence in a way that resonates with those who provide care and service to patients on a daily basis and (2) illustrate that excellent customer service makes their job easier? Without a way to create a widely shared understanding that service excellence works for them—as well as the patient—meaningful and lasting change is unlikely to occur.

How *Not* to Communicate the Initiative

We have all seen signs posted at the grocery store or on light poles asking for help in finding lost pets. But you might have missed this one:

Lost!

Small brown dog
Partially blind
One leg missing
Tail has been broken three times and hangs at an unusual angle
Recently neutered
Answers to the name "Lucky"

When you introduce customer service programs that do not clearly make your staff's job easier, they don't feel lucky—they feel *like* "Lucky"—they can't see, their tail has been broken, and they have been surgically altered. And they will want to know why they have to change. For highly trained professionals in particular, for whom asking "Why?" is an ingrained characteristic, "Because I said so" won't cut it. On the other hand, "Because this is an evidence-based discipline to make your job easier" works because there is a scientific base to support it.

A-TEAM MEMBERS VERSUS B-TEAM MEMBERS

The simplest way to communicate the belief that customer service behaviors actually make the job easier is to pose a single question to your healthcare providers: *Do we offer good customer service?*

Not surprisingly, typical answers include "Yes!" from some; an affirmative but less emphatic "yes"; and even the occasional "No, unfortunately, we don't offer consistently good customer service." In addition, a predictably large group will answer neither affirmatively nor negatively. They believe that the answer to the question is, "It depends." The next question, of course, is, "Upon *what* does it depend?" What are the factors that determine whether we offer good customer service? Again, a simple exercise serves us well in making this determination. Pose the following question to a healthcare team:

Do you sometimes look at the people you are working with and think to yourself, "Bring it on! Whatever we've got to do today, this team of people can make it happen!"?

Those individuals who proclaim "Yes!" are known as the A-Team. If you were to ask these folks to describe A-Team attributes and attitudes, their responses would likely include the following terms:

- Positive
- Proactive
- Confident
- Competent
- Trustworthy
- A teacher
- Does whatever it takes
- Compassionate
- A communicator
- A team player
- Has a sense of humor

This list summarizes the responses from the thousands of healthcare providers we've questioned about the attributes of the A-Team. Regardless of where they work in the healthcare system, the phenomenon of the A-Team is well known. This is a team we'd all like to work with—and join. These people make the hard work of providing patient care not only bearable but enjoyable. When you use this exercise, it is important to remember that you don't need to tell them what the A-Team attributes are (top down)—they already know and will tell you willingly (bottom up).

However, there is a second part to the above exercise that is equally, if not more, important. You now must ask the staff this question:

Do you sometimes look at the people you are working with and think
to yourself, "Shoot me, shoot me now! I can't work with him! Who in the world
makes the schedule around here?!"?

Those staff who make you think, "That's exactly how I feel" are B-Team players—also a well-known phenomenon among healthcare providers. B-Team members can be described in the following terms:

- Negative
- Reactive
- Confused
- A poor communicator
- Lazy
- Late
- Has a victim mentality

- Administrator Scrooge
- A constant complainer
- Can't do
- Always surprised
- Nurse Ratched
- Dr. Torquemada

Almost every institution has a Nurse Ratched, the quintessentially dour and negative nurse of Ken Kesey's *One Flew over the Cuckoo's Nest.* Many of you are also painfully aware that most institutions have their Dr. Torquemada, the Grand Inquisitor of the Spanish Inquisition. Nurses know that one B-Team doctor can extract more pain from the staff with his negative attitude in an eight-hour shift than Tomas Torquemada did in eight years of the Inquisition because doctors typically set the tone on the "attitude meter" by their actions. Unfortunately, your staff may also think you have an Administrator Scrooge on your management team. An important insight is to recognize that not only do all of you know who the Nurse Ratcheds, Dr. Torquemadas, and Administrator Scrooges are in your institutions but you also know their negative behaviors and faults in infinite detail.

In our seminars, we hear about a curious but predictable phenomenon whereby staff enjoy articulating the attributes that typify the A-Team but they truly delight in delineating the B-Team behaviors, often shouting them out, laughing as they do so. Regardless of the location where the service is provided, all members of a particular team understand on a fundamental level the phenomenon of the A-Team and the B-Team in their daily work. They also understand the toxic nature of the B-Team behaviors, as evidenced by their response to the question, "How many B-Team members does it take to destroy an entire shift?" Without exception, every audience shouts the same response—"One!"

How can this possibly be? Can a single person destroy the morale of your entire staff in a busy, clinical environment? You bet—and he or she does so daily and predictably in your hospital or healthcare institution. You know it, and, far more importantly, your staff know it—they know who these people are, precisely how they act, and the details of their toxic behavior.

Why Are B-Teams Problematic?

As one nursing director on a busy clinical unit in an academic medical center told us, "I don't really mind taking care of the patients; they're the reason I went into nursing and management in the first place. It's taking care of the B-Team members that wears me out. I don't know how much longer I can do it."

The fundamental problem with B-Team members is not that their behaviors create customer dissatisfaction (although they clearly and predictably do) or that they are harming patients (often, they know precisely where the line is between getting fired for patient negligence or malpractice and getting away with delivering poor customer service). The problem is that their actions and attitudes systematically demoralize the remainder of the healthcare team. A nursing director of a neurological unit, for example, tartly observed that "B-Team members are like space-occupying lesions—they take up space and drain energy." B-Team members foment discontent and nurture it in others. Thinking of the B-Team from the neurological perspective, the overall impact of its members on others is not neutral—it's not just that they lack the A-Team skills but also that they suck energy out of the system routinely.

If for no other reason, eliminating B-Team behaviors is essential to ensuring that employee satisfaction and morale are maintained at the highest possible level under the admittedly difficult circumstances faced in hospitals and healthcare systems.

Many B-Team members seem to be negative, reactive people who begin their day unhappy—and get unhappier by the minute, dragging the morale of patients and staff down with them. Why does this happen? How can people go to work, day after day, year after year, under such circumstances? Quite simply, *the B-Team members are doing a job that isn't their job to do.*

By this we mean that the B-Team members have, through multiple pathways and circumstances, ended up doing something for which they are not basically suited; they simply do not have the skills and abilities (largely from an interpersonal standpoint) required to do their job.

One of us (TM) is the father of three young men and, while the analogies between child rearing and leadership and management can certainly be overdrawn, this story is pertinent to both. Each morning when I dropped my sons off at school when they were younger, they heard the same thing from Dad: *One more step in the journey of discovering where your deep joy intersects the world's deep needs.*

(Understandably, they preferred to take the bus.) Nonetheless, the consistent message is to begin with "your deep joy" as opposed to the "world's deep needs," since all of us must discover what it is we enjoy doing, where it is we enjoy doing it, the kinds of people we enjoy doing it with, and the circumstances under which all of this occurs.

For people to become a doctor or nurse or healthcare executive because "the world needs them" is not a great idea. To become a doctor or a nurse or a healthcare executive to fulfill the fundamental joy they derive from serving people in need is a better match of the deep joy/deep need ratio. Many B-Team members have signed on for a job that is simply not their job to do. They would be better suited either in some other area of healthcare or in an altogether different area of the workforce.

For B-Team members, somehow the world is always a surprise to them—they are surprised that there are patients to be taken care of; they are surprised that these patients have needs and expectations that often do not match their own; they are surprised that available resources are taxed to provide such care; they are surprised by . . . *everything*. One emergency department medical director summed it up nicely:

> I don't understand how these people can be surprised. Many of them have been working in our emergency department for ten years. We see 75,000 visits in a space designed for 40,000, so it is a crazy place. These people have come to work every day for ten years and yet continue to ask, "Where in the world do all these people come from?" I always tell them, "I need to explain something to you. There is a big red sign above our door that says EMERGENCY, and it has an arrow pointing right at us. I think maybe that's where these people came from."

In this respect, B-Team members remind us of bobblehead dolls—they just stand there with a vacuous stare, their heads nodding vacantly to any question asked of them. However, A-Team members are rarely surprised, since they have a clear expectation and essential knowledge of where their deep joy intersects the world's deep needs. And even when they are surprised, they adapt to the unanticipated situation remarkably well, expressing the feelings of one A-Team member: "What's my job description? It's to do whatever I have to do to get through the day, to help my patients, to help the people with whom I work. My job description? I guess it's 'Do whatever it takes.'" This is someone we want to work with!

In addition to the negativity and unhappiness B-Team members bring to the workplace, however, is an even deeper and more basic reason to address problems introduced by their presence: Everyone in every area of your institution knows who the Nurse Ratcheds and Dr. Torquemadas are—except, of course, for Nurse Ratched and Dr. Torquemada—and if you consistently fail to deal with those B-Teamers, as dictated by the law of unintended consequences, you are demonstrating to your staff that you are dishonest as a leader. Why? Because you allow a system to operate in which there are two sets of rules: one set for the A-Team members and a separate set for Nurse Ratched and Dr. Torquemada. Perhaps the best indicator of this situation is if you hear staff members say some variant of the following:

"Oh, that's Dr. Smith—you have to learn how to deal with him."

"One more thing—when you work with Mr. Jones, he is always 'loaded for bear.' "

"Listen, Christine is a good nurse, but she can be really prickly."

All of these comments are signs that a dishonest double standard is in place, and your reputation will pay the price for it if you don't aggressively and visibly correct the problems related to the B-Team.

We offer several detailed strategies on how to deal with the B-Team in Chapter 9. For now, suffice to note that one of the most important outcomes of a successful customer service program that addresses and eliminates B-Team behaviors is that A-Team members who have tolerated B-Team members' behavior for years will understand that leadership and management are *finally* serious about systematically addressing the problem. If you deal with your Nurse Ratched and Dr. Torquemada, your staff will understand that something is different about *this* customer service program—that people will be held accountable for service *and* disservice.

> A-Team behaviors = good customer service . . . *and employee satisfaction*
>
> B-Team behaviors = bad customer service . . . *and employee dissatisfaction*

They're Still Here?

It's not hard to see the damage that B-Teams do to the delivery of healthcare and the healing environment. So why haven't we gotten rid of the B-Team members? Again, posing a simple query to the staff helps gain insight into this issue:

Are you an A-Team member?

Most people to whom this question is posed answer, "Of course, darn right, I am an A-Team member and very proud of it!" (It is a curious comment on human nature that few people ever admit, "I am a B-Team member with 20 years of providing miserable service.")

When A-Team members look in the mirror, what do they see? They see an A-Team member, since these people tend to be self-aware and have a clear understanding of what works and what doesn't work, both in the workplace and in their private lives. They know what their A-Team behaviors are and how to apply them, even if that understanding is, to a certain extent, on the subconscious level.

When B-Team members look in the mirror, what do they see? B-Team members see an A-Team member in the reflection, since they do not recognize that their attitudes and behaviors have a poisonous effect on those around them. (B-Team members are worse than vampires—vampires don't see *any* reflection, whereas B-Team members see the *opposite* of reality.) For B-Team members, their behaviors and attitudes work—for them.

One role of leadership and management is, with the assistance of the A-Team, to *hold the mirror up to the B-Team members,* letting them see the impact that their behavior has on patients, families, and other members of the healthcare team.

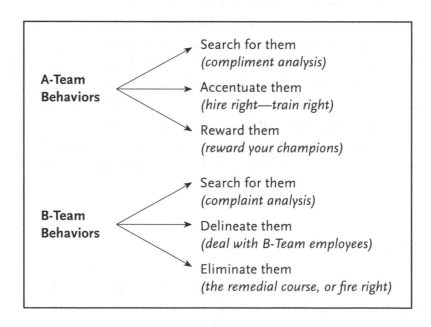

CHANGING BEHAVIOR: INTRINSIC VERSUS EXTRINSIC CHANGE

One basic truth of the human condition is that

All meaningful and lasting change is intrinsically motivated.

While extrinsic change may produce immediate results, those results plateau quickly before decaying steadily over time. Natural diffusion of change—intrinsically generated—takes longer to result in a positive alteration of behavior, but it is more sustainable and exceeds the impact of extrinsic motivation, as seen in Exhibit 1.1.

Effecting intrinsic change ("It makes your job easier") instead of extrinsic change ("Get your scores up because I am the boss and I said so!") results in shifting the effectiveness of change dramatically to the left of the scale shown in Exhibit 1.1, both accelerating the pace of change and sustaining its effectiveness over time, as seen in Exhibit 1.2.

To be sure, extrinsic motivation is seductive. It draws us in by appealing to our desire to mandate immediate change. Watch George C. Scott's mesmerizing and Oscar-winning performance in *Patton,* and you will see a good example of how some bosses act—storming around giving commands. But the real George S. Patton was a far more complex and effective leader, one who understood the importance of being at the front lines so the troops knew their leader was with them—an early version of rounding (discussed in detail in Chapter 11). He also made the connection between motivation and execution (Blumenson 1996):

Exhibit 1.1: Extrinsic Change Versus Natural Change

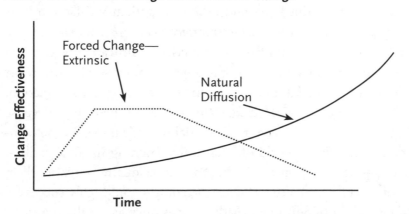

Exhibit 1.2: Extrinsic Change Versus Intrinsic Change

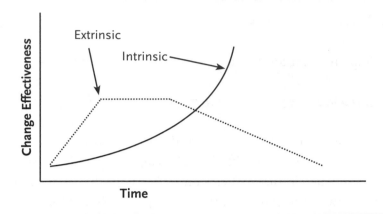

It comes down to using intrinsic motivation to drive execution. *Without the ability to execute, all other attributes of leadership become hollow and meaningless.* (Emphasis added.)

Execution is also discussed in chapters 6 and 8. For now, suffice to say that execution requires the *specificity* of clear goals and objectives, widely known and shared throughout the organization, as well as the *sensitivity* of using intrinsic motivation to achieve self-motivation in professionals to move toward change—particularly nonincremental change.

INTRODUCTION TO THE SURVIVAL SKILLS

The biggest difference between this book and others on patient satisfaction is its basic tenet: *The number one reason to get customer service right is that it makes the job easier.* As illustrated by the A-Team and B-Team exercises, healthcare providers can clearly see that A-Team behaviors are also high-value customer service behaviors that improve not only patient and family satisfaction but also employee satisfaction.

We call these behaviors our *Survival Skills*. Why do we call them that? Because the skill set that supports A-Team behavior is essential to our survival in the complex, complicated, and confusing world of healthcare. Training in these skills—or A-Team behaviors—is an investment in the most precious resource in all of healthcare: the providers of care. Herb Kelleher, the colorful and highly successful cofounder and former CEO of Southwest Airlines, was once asked the question, "If you had to choose, would you invest in the employee or in the customer?" His answer came instantly: "In the employee! Because if you take care of the employees, they'll take care of the customers" (Frieberg and Frieberg 1996).

In the remainder of this book, we discuss the importance of understanding expectations (Chapter 2), define the patient–customer axis (Chapter 3), share our Survival Skills (chapters 4–6), and break down the tools in the A-Team Tool Kit and how to apply them (chapters 7–17).

CONCLUSION

Peter Drucker (2010) notes that all service businesses require the voluntary contribution of the provider to choose the type of service that will be created in the interaction with the customer. Therefore, according to Drucker, all service workers are "volunteers." You cannot force your employees—much less the physicians with whom you work—to be nice, professional, friendly, and caring. However, you can show them that all efforts to provide excellent customer service make their job easier, and all successful customer service initiatives recognize this fundamental truth and put it to work effectively.

SURVIVAL SKILLS SUMMARY

While the CEO's and senior management's commitment to customer service is essential, your staff has to understand the following:

- The number one reason to get customer service right is that it makes the job easier.
- The customer service litmus test is that if an action or a decision doesn't make the job easier for your staff, it isn't *really* customer service.
- The A-Team is a group of people who are admired and respected because their behaviors and attributes make life easier, not just for the patient but also for those with whom they work.
- Discover who the A-Team members are in your organization and learn what they are doing.
- Use the A-Team/B-Team exercise to demonstrate to your staff that A-Team behaviors are simply good customer service that will make their jobs easier.
- The B-Team members' attitudes and attributes make life miserable for the patient and your staff. Discovering who the B-Team members are is, strangely, much easier than identifying the A-Team members.

- How many B-Team members does it take to destroy an entire shift? One!
- Identify A-Team members and the skills they use—then accentuate them, insist on them, and reward them.
- Identify B-Team members and behaviors—then eliminate either the behaviors or the people. No less than your integrity is at stake.
- Identify your Nurse Ratched, Dr. Torquemada, and Administrator Scrooge— let them know it's time to get with the program or get gone.
  - Use a combination of specificity and sensitivity—intrinsic motivation—to drive execution.

REFERENCES

Argyris, C. 1993. *Knowledge for Action: A Guide to Overcoming Barriers to Organizational Change.* San Francisco: Jossey-Bass.

Belasco, J. A., and R. C. Stayer. 1993. *The Flight of the Buffalo.* New York: Warner Books.

Blumenson, M. 1996. *The Patton Papers.* New York: Houghton-Mifflin.

Collins, J. 2010. *How the Mighty Fall: And Why Some Never Give In.* New York: HarperCollins.

Drucker, P. 2010. *Drucker on Leadership.* San Francisco: Jossey-Bass.

Frieberg, K., and J. Frieberg. 1996. *Nuts! Southwest Airlines' Crazy Recipe for Business and Personal Success.* New York: Bard Press.

Hickson, G. 2009. "Discouraging Disruptive Behavior: It Starts with a Cup of Coffee!" PowerPoint presentation. Accessed August 20, 2013. www .studergroupmedia.com/WRIHC2009/presentations/discouraging_ disruptive_behavior_it_starts_with_a_cup_of_coffee_vandy_hickson.pdf.

MORE RESOURCES ON CUSTOMER SERVICE

Berry, L. L. 1999. *Discovering the Soul of Service: The Nine Drivers of Sustainable Business Success.* New York: Free Press.

Berry, L. L., and K. D. Seltman. 2008. *Leadership Lessons from Mayo Clinic: Inside One of the World's Most Admired Service Organizations.* New York: McGraw-Hill.

Len Berry is the preeminent source concerning the science of service. This study of 14 service industry leaders has many lessons for healthcare.

Block, P. 2002. *The Right Use of Power: How Stewardship Replaces Leadership.* Louisville, CO: Sounds True.

Audio/CD available at PeterBlock.com.

Patterson, K., J. Grenny, R. McMillan, A. Switzler, and S. Covey. 2002. *Crucial Conversations: Tools for Talking When the Stakes Are High.* New York: McGraw-Hill.

Peters, T. 2010. *The Little Big Things: 163 Ways to Pursue Excellence.* New York: Harper Business.

The latest from the incomparable Tom Peters—a great resource and a great read.

CHAPTER 2

Understanding Expectations

We have shown that the first step in the journey to service excellence is to establish the "why," which is to make the difficult and demanding job of healthcare delivery easier. That is precisely why patient satisfaction and employee satisfaction are as inextricably bound as clinical and service excellence. The sentiment behind great customer service is "both/and," never "either/or." Service excellence in healthcare is therefore an evidence-based discipline, designed to be used to deliver predictable and positive results.

In *The Fifth Discipline,* Peter Senge (2006) argues persuasively that all of us carry certain "mental models," or sets of beliefs and understandings about certain issues. These mental models combine to form the lens through which we view the problems and opportunities we face. *Understanding expectations* is a key mental model for improving service in healthcare.

EXPECTATIONS FOR GREAT CUSTOMER SERVICE

In each clinical situation in the healthcare environment, from treating the most acutely ill or severely injured patient to conducting the simplest outpatient laboratory test, the patients, their families, and their loved ones bring a certain set of expectations to the encounter. We call these *expectation packets.* They essentially form the patient's mental model of what is anticipated to transpire over the course of the healthcare encounter, and they must be unbundled or unpacked if we are to know what is within them. To be clear, these expectations can be accurate or inaccurate, but they must never be ignored.

One of the central problems in healthcare service is that many providers and staff in healthcare feel it is their job to simply meet patients' expectations—no more and no less. But if the healthcare system does no more than meet expectations, the encounter goes as expected and the patient is "merely satisfied."

Patient/family expectations met ➤ *merely satisfied*

In other words, such staff are "just enoughers"—people who are doing just enough to meet expectations and thus keep their jobs. Rather than having poor character, however, these B-Team members have not been educated to accept excellence over adequacy.

In our current highly competitive and capacity-constrained healthcare market, is *merely satisfied* good enough? No way—much more than "merely" is needed to meet or exceed the targets being set. And who wants to lead a team of people who wake up in the morning and say, "I can't *wait* to get out there and be the 50th percentile!"? To put mere adequacy in perspective, think about these questions:

If you rank at the 50th percentile as the result of your performance on a test, is that a passing grade or a failing grade?

If someone were drowning 20 feet from shore and you threw him or her a rope 11 feet long, how likely would you be to save that person?

Just-enoughers simply are not enough to get by with anymore. Our boards and leadership teams can no longer accept the *mean*—it is excellence we seek, and it is difficult, if not impossible, to create staff satisfaction if we are OK with merely satisfying our patients. To be sure, if your patient satisfaction scores are in the 15th percentile, moving to the 50th percentile is on the path to the top, but it should just be a temporary stop on that path.

FAILING TO MEET EXPECTATIONS: THE ORIGINS OF COMPLAINTS

When a patient's or family's expectations are not met, that customer is dissatisfied and may complain. The extent of the difference between patients' expectations and the failure to deliver on those expectations dictates the focus of the resulting complaint.

Healthcare professionals may feel that the patient's or family's expectations were unreasonable or too high, but this sentiment ignores the critical importance of negotiating expectations, which is a bedrock skill for everyone in healthcare, as we discuss in detail in Chapter 5. Examples of complaints abound, and we have heard them all, from timeliness of care to cleanliness of the environment to attitudes of the staff to the level of communication . . . you get the picture.

Think about your own customer service experiences. When you see dirty trays and seats on an airline, you can't help but wonder how well the maintenance crews are servicing the engines or how attentive the ground crews are at getting luggage to the right destination. Patients are equally attentive—and equally adept at extrapolating from an issue of dirty linen to one of poor clinical care. These are all "quality surrogates." They are not, strictly speaking, markers or metrics that indicate quality, but they are elements that patients, families, and even staff view as surrogate measures of the organization's commitment to excellence.

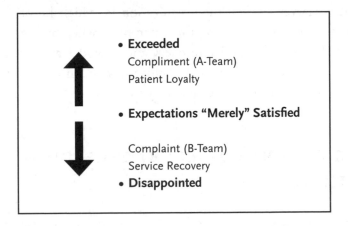

To demonstrate this relationship, we share the unfortunate experience that I (TM) had with one of my sons, Josh (about whom you will hear more later). Josh was diagnosed with a 3-centimeter basilar artery aneurysm. Virtually every medical center in the world told us it was an inoperable lesion. But Dr. Robert Spetzler and his team at Barrow Neurological Institute in Phoenix had a solution. When we arrived at the institute, we found the facilities to be, let's say, Spartan—clean, but minimal in the creature comforts and certainly not luxurious. As soon as we arrived, a nurse told us, "At Barrow, we invest our dollars in having the best staff available—and we have the best in the world. If the 'hotel' part of our experience is not Ritz-Carlton, trust us, the medical and nursing care is." At some level, perception *is* reality, but *managing* that perception is within range for all of us if we make it a part of an evidence-based discipline to meet expectations.

Josh's surgery—among the most risky and complicated procedures in all of neurosurgery—went perfectly, so well in fact that he not only survived but now has a lovely wife, Valerie, and two wonderful daughters, Eve and Audra. While we were at Barrow, we never complained about the conditions; in fact, seeing the state of the facility made us smile to think how great the doctors and nurses were. Each year we cheerfully send a modest donation to Barrow, and we know where the investment will go.

The point is simple, obvious, and vastly underappreciated: Not every healthcare institution is blessed with great capital resources, but all of us can apply the evidence-based discipline of meeting expectations in full and helping patients and families understand how we use what resources we do have.

Whenever we discover that expectations are not being met, the skill of service recovery must be used to rectify the situation as fast as possible. When should this occur? The instant we realize that we have failed to meet a patient's or family's expectations. Who should perform service recovery activities? Whoever identifies the failure, at whatever level of the organization in which he or she resides. Of course, it is also important to have a protocol in place whereby a leader or manager is informed of the need for service recovery and provides appropriate follow-up, but every person should be trained to recognize service failures and initiate service recovery. Chapter 8 describes service recovery in detail.

CREATING PATIENT LOYALTY BY EXCEEDING EXPECTATIONS

Even if the staff have not been trained in the concept of expectation packets and how failing to deliver on patients' expectations creates the need for service recovery, once they are introduced to it, they will quickly recognize this philosophical construct and how it can make their job easier. However, it takes time for them to understand what follows—often to their surprise: Loyal patients are created who "sing the praises" of your institution and the staff who provided their care simply because those patients were provided a service that was better than expected.

Such patients are in many ways the Holy Grail of healthcare service, for reasons detailed later. Many people working in healthcare can recall a great story about a patient who expressed his or her gratitude and respect for the care and comfort provided. Often, it's the fuel that keeps us going.

I (RC) frequently tell the story of 60-year-old Ed Corwin (not his real name), who lived in a small southwestern Virginia community located more than 300 miles from the National Cancer Institute (NCI) in Bethesda, Maryland. Ed had been newly diagnosed with small cell lung cancer and, because of the dismal prognosis at that time, had been referred to the NCI for treatment. All of his treatment, both inpatient and outpatient, was conducted at the NCI, and because Ed's outpatient clinic session was at 8:00 a.m., he and his wife would get up before 3:00 a.m. to drive the 300 miles to Bethesda. During the course of his treatment, a bond formed between Ed, his wife, and me such that we looked forward to seeing each other in spite of the surrounding radiation therapy and chemotherapy. One particular winter morning, as we greeted each other, Mrs. Corwin said, "Dr. C, when we left this morning I had some good homemade biscuits for you and some country ham." I soon learned that "had" was the key word, as she continued, "But we hadn't gone more than 20 miles from home before Ed got to smelling it and ate it all." I looked over at Ed, and he gave me the biggest grin you ever saw.

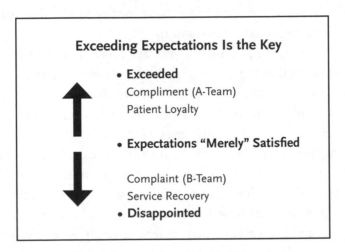

During the time he was a patient at the NCI, we gave Ed the best treatment available in the United States, and he accepted it with grace and equanimity (with the help of his lovely wife). Eventually, he passed away. Usually the death of a patient signals the end of the doctor–patient relationship, but Mrs. Corwin taught me otherwise. She continued to call me at the NIH after Ed's death. On one of those occasions I finally "got it" when she said, "You know, Dr. C, I call you because I think he is still there with you." I learned at that moment that the *science* often does not outlive the patient encounter, no matter how good it was, but the *art* often outlives the patient. Surviving relatives retell the stories of positive interactions with their caregivers, and we caregivers retell stories of bonds formed, patients who became part of us, and biscuits that never quite made it to the table.

So exceeding expectations occurs in areas beyond clinical quality—and in those realms it can have even more far-reaching effects. One of the first and best voices to discuss the concept of customer loyalty was that of Frederick Reichheld (1996), of Bain & Company. His work was credited with providing a clear lens through which to view the role of exceeding expectations in service industries.

Unhappy customers tell an average of 20 to 25 people about their bad experience. These data originally came from the Technical Assistance Research Project and reflected non-healthcare experience, but this finding has become "lore" in healthcare. It has a pernicious impact in that staff—and some managers—can generate an attitude of "What can you do? We can't win with odds like that." But what healthcare leaders and managers need to know and widely disseminate is an even more astounding statistic: Customers whose expectations have been exceeded tell an average of *40 to 50 people* how happy they were with their experience. There are few "magic bullets" in life, but this is one of them. Leaders who understand, promote, and advance the concept of patient loyalty hold substantial leverage in dramatically improving patient satisfaction.

Sometimes the most important insights are those that are the most obvious. The concept of strengthening patient loyalty by taking a systematic approach to understanding and exceeding expectations in healthcare is a simple one. Giving organizations the vision and tools to do so also makes staff's and clinicians' lives easier—fulfilling the "why" of healthcare service excellence.

Tolstoy recognized this wisdom in the opening line of *Anna Karenina*: "Happy families are all alike; each unhappy family is unhappy in its own way." The same is true for patient loyalty. All loyal patients are satisfied and recognize, tacitly if not explicitly, that their expectations have been exceeded, whereas each unsatisfied, nonloyal patient has his own issue that he feels strongly about. When you start to hear patients express the following sentiment, you'll know patient loyalty is rising: "I don't know what's going on at Memorial Hospital, but they are really getting it right over there!"

Chapter 4 discusses in more detail the ways in which we can make the customer service diagnosis and offer the right treatment. Chapter 12 explores the importance of using scripts—evidence-based language—to ensure that we not only exceed patients' and families' expectations but also educate them to recognize when their expectations have been exceeded. For the moment, suffice to say that gaining a common understanding throughout the US healthcare system about patients' expectations lays the foundation for increasing satisfaction and making staff's jobs easier.

CONCLUSION

We diagnose and treat various diseases as a fundamental part of our work in healthcare. It is time we understood fully that we also need to recruit and retain individuals whom we can train and encourage to diagnose patients' and families' expectations.

SURVIVAL SKILLS SUMMARY

- The "why" of achieving service excellence is that it makes our jobs easier.
- Improving customer service starts with gaining an understanding that patients and their families come to the healthcare experience with a set of expectations, or an expectation packet.
- If we simply meet the patients' expectations, they are merely satisfied, meaning they are neither disappointed nor delighted.
- If we fail to meet expectations as a result of B-Team behaviors or processes, patients are unhappy, which is the source of complaints.
- Navigating patients' expectations is a core competency for members of the healthcare team.
- Exceeding expectations through A-Team behaviors and processes leads to patient loyalty, which is a very powerful force in healthcare.
- Whereas unhappy patients tell about 20 people of their bad experience, loyal patients tell 40 to 50 people how delighted they were with their encounter.

REFERENCES

Reichheld, F. 1996. *The Loyalty Effect: The Hidden Force Behind Growth, Profits, and Lasting Value*. Boston: Harvard Business School Press.

Senge, P. 2006. *The Fifth Discipline: The Art and Practice of the Learning Organization*. New York: Doubleday.

CHAPTER 3

Are They Patients, or Are They Customers?

As healthcare organizations increasingly take responsibility for creating a culture of organization-wide accountability, one of the most important and difficult tasks is to develop a concise and meaningful answer to the question regarding the people in your care: *Are they patients, or are they customers?*

The majority of physicians, nurses, and healthcare workers whom we have encountered in our practice and research indicate that the answer to this question is straightforward—individuals seeking care are patients, not customers. Common reactions include:

"This is not Nordstrom or Wal-Mart—they are patients, not customers."

"Stop calling them patients? Start calling them customers? Give me a break! Better yet, give me some medication for my nausea."

"We're not here to practice McDonald's medicine."

Resistance to the concept of patients as customers is understandable, if frustrating for healthcare management. And the more acute the healthcare setting is, the more dramatic the resistance is. Years ago, as emergency physicians, we thought it was a good idea to buy our emergency department (ED) nurses T-shirts that read: "I'm here to save your butt, Not Kiss It!"

We thought it was hilarious. How were we supposed to know they would wear them to work? And how were we supposed to know the CEO would pick that day to round in the ED? Trust us—she was not amused. It took us months to recover her trust and respect from that debacle.

Your clinical staff clearly see those they care for as patients. But are they customers as well? *Customers* could refer to a diverse range of participants in the healthcare process, including patients; family members; payers; employers; and the providers of healthcare themselves, who are internal customers to the process. However, for the purposes of our discussion, let's restrict the use of the term to those who are the direct recipients of the healthcare provided.

So, what are they? To stimulate discussion of this question, we use an exercise to tease out healthcare professionals' own inherent and intuitive definitions of customers and patients. We ask them to imagine a gauge with a needle that will point toward either "patient" or "customer," depending solely on their reactions to specific clinical scenarios (see Exhibit 3.1).

Following are three clinical scenarios drawn from the ED. (Appendix 3.1 offers scenarios from other healthcare settings.) After reading each scenario, we pose the simple question, "Is this a patient or a customer?"

Scenario 1. A 65-year-old woman presents to the ED with severe, crushing, substernal chest pain that began 30 minutes earlier. The patient rates her pain as a 9 on a scale of 10, which is unrelieved by the nitroglycerine given by the paramedics en route. Her EKG (electrocardiograph) clearly shows an acute anterior myocardial infarction. *Is this a patient or a customer?*

Scenario 2. A three-year-old child presents to the ED at 3 o'clock in the morning, having been seen by his pediatrician at 3 o'clock in the afternoon, where a diagnosis of an ear infection was made, the patient was started on antibiotics, and the parents were given fever control instructions. Now the patient has a temperature of 99.2°F (normal being 98.6°F) and the parents say they "can't get the fever down," despite

---

Exhibit 3.1: The Patient–CustoMeter

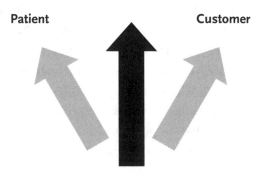

Patient   Customer

---

the fact that the parents have not followed the fever reduction instructions and the antibiotic prescription hasn't been filled. *Is this a patient or a customer?*

Scenario 3. Same as Scenario 2, with one exception—the child is your own. *Is this a patient or a customer?*

We have posed these questions to thousands of healthcare professionals from diverse backgrounds living in a variety of geographic locations, and the results are absolutely consistent: The woman in scenario 1 is universally described as a patient, whereas the child in scenario 2 is described as a customer (with the parents being identified as the primary customer). Scenario 3 invariably causes healthcare professionals to question whether they would classify their own child as a patient or a customer. As we hear from many respondents, "The needle wavers a little on that third scenario." When asked why they rate the woman as a patient and the child (and his parents) as customers, the results are also highly predictable, as characterized in Exhibit 3.2.

Patients are considered more acutely ill or injured, feel quite sick, have little or no choice in where they seek their healthcare, and are largely dependent on the healthcare practitioner to deliver technical expertise in a time-dependent fashion. In patient–clinician relationships, the healthcare professional is the primary locus of power and has control during the clinical encounter.

Customers are seen as less acutely ill or injured, have substantial choice in where their healthcare is provided, are more independent, and have substantially more

Exhibit 3.2: Clinicians' General Characterizations of Patients Versus Customers

Patient	Customer
Is acutely ill or injured	Is less severely ill
Is dependent on physician	Is independent
Power/control lies with clinician	Power/control lies with customer
Has less choice	Has more choice
Technical expertise is required	Service skills are required
Higher satisfaction is experienced by clinician	Lower satisfaction is experienced by clinician
High clarity of treatment is required	Less clarity of treatment is required
Encounter is time dependent	Encounter is service dependent

power and control over the healthcare encounter than do patients. The needs of customers are more service dependent, while those of patients are more clinically dependent.

It is important to note that healthcare professionals tell us without exception that they feel a high degree of clarity in knowing how to take care of patients, who primarily require technical expertise to treat their illnesses or injuries. However, most healthcare professionals are far less clear about how to approach customers, largely because providers lack specific and detailed training in addressing a customer's needs and expectations.

The earlier exercise helps your staff recognize that they subconsciously and tacitly ask the question, "Is this a patient or a customer?" every time they pick up a patient's chart. And they make that determination by using a simple, straightforward, but unwritten diagnostic rule known intuitively to everyone in healthcare:

> *The more horizontal they are, the more they're patients.*
> *The more vertical they are, the more they're customers.*

This rule has virtually 100 percent sensitivity and specificity—in other words, it never fails. Those who are horizontal (or nearly so)—they are unable to sit up on their own—are dependent on the delivery of technical skills, often in an expert and rapid fashion. Those who are more vertical—they can sit up independently—have more control in the provider–patient/customer relationship and are often unafraid to exercise that control, sometimes to the consternation of the healthcare provider.

HIGH VERSUS LOW EXPECTATIONS

Our research indicates that the role of expectations is a crucial one in healthcare, as we indicate in Chapter 2. To illustrate, we ask course participants, "Who has higher expectations—the lady with the heart attack or the parents of the child with a fever?" The answer is always "the parents." What are the parents' (customers') expectations? They want reassurance that their child is not acutely ill so that they can go home, put the child to bed, and get back to sleep. What is it that the lady (patient) wants? Well, she wants to live.

Let's make sure that we have this right: The parents want fever control instructions and reassurance so they can sleep. In general, staff consider that desire to constitute "high expectations." The lady is dying and wants treatment so she continues to live. Providers typically consider that desire to fall under the "low expectations" category. Intuitively, this mentality seems odd. How can someone who is dying have low expectations? How can giving reassurance to parents be a high expectation? Is this fundamentally flawed reasoning?

No, because what that lady is "buying"—lifesaving care—is what providers love to "sell" and are *highly trained* in its delivery. Providers enjoy taking care of patients who are that severely ill because it is a skill in which they have a high degree of confidence. Saving lives—that's what they signed up for!

The parents' expectation—reassurance that the child is OK—is not part of the curriculum for our medical schools or nursing schools, and our healthcare institutions generally don't address it well in orientation or in-service programs. (Duke University School of Medicine, where we teach our service excellence program as a part of its capstone course, represents at least one exception to the rule.) Providers have not been explicitly trained to meet customers' expectations in a detailed, evidence-based fashion. Further, such expectations seem high because clinicians do not derive nearly as much satisfaction from giving fever control instructions as from saving lives. That shouldn't be surprising—Maslow's hierarchy of needs might suggest that the path to self-actualization for most healthcare professionals is more easily attained through lifesaving interventions than patient education.

IMPORTANCE OF LANGUAGE IN THE HEALTHCARE JOURNEY

Is the job to care or to cure? Is it the journey or the destination? We travel the country speaking about customer service. How much credit do you think we give the airlines for getting us from point A to point B and not crashing the plane? How about *none*—we expect to land safely. Your patients expect excellent clinical care (the destination). But they also expect excellent service (the journey). The destination is assumed; the journey is usually how service is judged.

Take the "Are they patients, or are they customers?" exercise further by asking, "During a typical day at your job, how many patients do you see, and how many customers?" Even in a busy ED or trauma/critical care unit, it is not uncommon to hear ratios of 80 to 90 percent customers and 10 to 20 percent patients (see Exhibit 3.3). If that is your staff's perception (and it clearly is), then the following is also true:

The sicker the patient is, the better the providers like him.

Exhibit 3.3: The Patient–CustoMeter Rule

Patient

Customer
90%
These people are the <u>price</u> we pay . . .

. . . for the privilege of taking care of these
10%

Most providers go into healthcare to make a difference in people's lives—that is their "deep joy and deep need." What nurse is really enthused about a fully ambulatory "customer" who hits the call light every 17 seconds? A tremendous amount of job and personal satisfaction comes from caring for those who are severely ill and injured and somewhat less for those with high expectations that are often also seen as unreasonable.

So which is it, are they patients, or are they customers? Is it the art or the science that we practice? Is it the name ("Mrs. Gazungas in room 4") or the disease ("The belly pain in room 5")? At one academic medical center with an international reputation, we overheard a resident say to one of her colleagues, "I just saw your appendix." Now, either she had flunked anatomy or she had seen a *patient* with suspected appendicitis. *All language has meaning.* Therefore, language in your institution should reflect the commitment to the patient, not the disease.

GOOD PATIENTS?

After the "Are they patients, or are they customers?" exercise, we also ask the staff to help us define what, in their minds, constitutes a "good patient." It might surprise—or shock—you to learn that the responses we get throughout the country are summarized as follows:

- Is in restraints
- Is gagged
- Is handcuffed
- Is an orphan (has no family)
- Is compliant (wants it "our" way)

- Speaks "our" language
- Doesn't come back
- Is in and out fast
- Wants only one thing

The restriction-related responses speak to how much we prefer patients to customers. And then there's the orphan remark. No family? Great, except, of course, when it comes time to discharge them—and then we only want one family member around, and we prefer not to have to talk to her. At times it seems Nurse Ratched and Dr. Torquemada would leave patients on the ramp with discharge instructions pinned to their chest to avoid speaking to the family. As a staff member at one organization told us, "You have to understand—families complicate things."

The one adjective that is mentioned by every audience we speak to is *compliant*. When we ask attendees what that means, they say, "It means that they do what they're told; they follow directions."

If This Were Your Business . . .

If your staff's list of responses to the question, "What makes a good patient?" is similar to the one above (and it will be), it is important to make an additional point:

> *What if this were not healthcare but your own business,*
> *your own entrepreneurial venture? How would you define good?*

Ask your staff to imagine the following:

The organization is giving each of you an entrepreneurial venture. Your entire future, your retirement, your benefits, your salary, your savings plan, and your ability to send your kids to college depend on the success of that venture.

The entrepreneurial venture is a chicken franchise called Bucket O'Clucks. What factors would guide the success of your chicken franchise? Now, compare your customer requirements to what you told us constitutes good patients.

"In restraints, gagged, and handcuffed" wouldn't make any sense at all (unless your chicken franchise was serving incarcerates). If you have a chicken franchise, you don't want orphans because you want them to bring the entire family. How about "Speaks 'our' language"? In your chicken franchise, you don't care what language they speak—they can point to the chicken. "Doesn't come back"? If it were your entrepreneurial venture, you would want them to come back for breakfast, lunch, and dinner. "In and out fast"? No, you would want them to linger and come back for seconds. "Wants only one thing"? Of course not. How about some side dishes with that chicken? And a nice slice of pie or cheesecake? Finally, "Compliant—wants it our way"? As Burger King once advertised, "Have it *your* way." The point is simple—if this were the staff's entrepreneurial venture, if their livelihoods completely depended on its performance, in many ways you would want the opposite of what, albeit with gallows humor, your staff might deem as good patients.

Now ask your staff how many years they have worked at your healthcare institution. Five years? Ten years? Fifteen years? Twenty years? More? How many hands go up to indicate more than ten years of service?

The punch line? "I have news for those of you who have worked here more than ten years—this *is* your chicken franchise." None will miss the point that this is a business that they need to grow and treat as their own entrepreneurial venture. Their futures *do* depend on the success of this enterprise. While they may not own it in the entrepreneurial sense, they "own it" in the sense that their futures, hopes, and deep joy are invested in its viability.

WHAT PERCENTAGE PATIENT, AND WHAT PERCENTAGE CUSTOMER?

Practical experience and common sense tell you what textbooks do not:

> *If someone is about 80 percent patient (horizontal),*
> *he is also about 20 percent customer (vertical).*

The relationship could be described in a graph, with the customer percentage on the vertical axis and the patient percentage on the horizontal as shown in Exhibit 3.4.

It's a fairly simple but straightforward concept: Percent patient + percent customer = 100 percent. The equation then begs the question, *Wouldn't it work well if we treated the percent patient with technical skills and the percent customer with customer service skills?*

Let's say we estimate that the child from scenario 2 (the three-year-old in the ED at 3:00 a.m.) is about 80 percent customer and about 20 percent patient. That ratio implies that we should treat the 80 percent customer with service skills (A-Team behaviors). It might sound like this:

Triage nurse: I have kids of my own, and I know how hard it can be when your child is ill. However, the good news is that his temperature is actually normal, so he doesn't have what we define medically as a fever, even though his head may feel hot to the touch. Let's have the doctor examine him, but it's very likely you'll be able to go home and get some rest once he's been evaluated and treated.

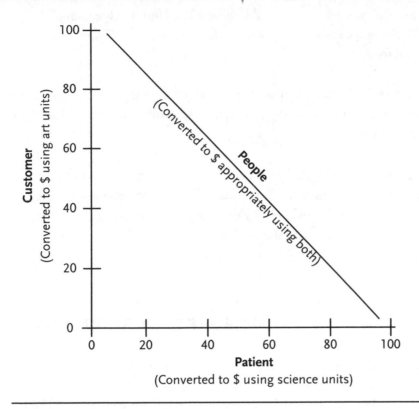

Combining the 80 percent customer with the 20 percent patient might sound like this:

> *Emergency physician:* I've examined your child very thoroughly, and I agree with your pediatrician that he has an ear infection, but I see no evidence of a more serious illness, such as meningitis. We should continue the fluids and the antibiotic and other medications you've been giving to control his temperature. You've done a great job, since his temperature is normal. We'll give him another dose of antibiotic to boost his blood level. Go home, get some rest, and I suggest calling your doctor in the morning. Do you have any questions?

For an ICU (intensive care unit) patient just out of surgery, the 90 percent patient conversation might go like this:

> *ICU nurse:* I know you are uncomfortable and the breathing tube is keeping you from talking, but we hope to take that out later today. Your vital signs are stable

and everything is proceeding the way we want it to. My priority is to keep it that way and to make sure you are as comfortable as possible. Until the breathing tube comes out, you can let me know what you need either with the call bell or by writing it on this pad for me.

For a patient who is in the second postoperative day following knee replacement surgery and beginning to ambulate (and therefore becoming more vertical), the dialogue might go as follows:

Medical/surgical floor nurse: Mrs. Rodriguez, you are progressing really well. You are actually ahead of where we expect you to be because you are walking much better and farther than most people at this stage. If we can help you maintain that progress, we may be able to get you home even sooner than we discussed. Today, the focus is on physical therapy, where Emily will be working with you.

A PREVIEW OF PART II AND THE FIRST SURVIVAL SKILL

One major problem with healthcare in the United States is that the system is often terrific at treating the patient/technical side of care delivery and poor at treating the customer/service side. An essential concept we present in our Survival Skills seminars is the necessity to understand the following:

> *Just as every patient receives a clinical diagnosis,*
> *she also should receive a customer service diagnosis.*

This tenet leads us to the first Survival Skill, which is the topic of the next chapter: *Make the customer service diagnosis (as well as the clinical diagnosis), and offer the right treatment.*

Nearly a century ago, Sir William Osler made a similar point: "It is more important to know what sort of patient has the disease than what sort of disease the patient has" (Cushing 1940). The patient–customer equation, while extremely helpful in understanding the customer service diagnosis, is not static. Although the formula is simple, as described earlier, it is not simply applied; your staff can't just make both the customer service diagnosis and the clinical diagnosis, treat both, and declare victory. As the patient journeys through the healthcare system, it is incumbent on you and your staff to ensure that she moves from the horizontal to the vertical. As that journey progresses, her needs change from those of a patient to those of a customer. When a patient presents to the ED in cardiac arrest, she is nearly 100 percent horizontal. Once the providers have resuscitated her and transferred her to the cardiac care unit, the patient–customer axis rotates as she becomes more vertical. When it's time for her discharge from the hospital, the patient has completed the journey to being nearly 100 percent vertical. To maintain awareness of patients' status, providers need to continue to ask themselves, *Has the patient– customer axis rotated today?*

In the inpatient setting—and to meaningful degrees in all of healthcare—we are in the business of taking patients from horizontal to vertical, from patients to customers, from dependent to independent. The patient with the knee replacement is quite horizontal on the day of surgery but becomes more vertical each subsequent day until discharge. The first day postoperatively sees caregivers more focused on pain control and prevention of deep vein thrombosis, but in subsequent days, as the patient becomes more upright, the focus changes to developing confidence in the patient's ability to ambulate. The elderly patient with community-acquired pneumonia may need ventilator assistance and ICU care and is thus horizontal on admission. But as her status improves and she becomes more vertical, she is increasingly ready for transfer to the medical/surgical floor.

> It is more important to know what sort of patient has the disease than what sort of disease the patient has.
> —Sir William Osler

From the patient's perspective, say a 55-year-old patient (male or female) has had three coronary artery stents placed. Initially, the patient is understandably concerned about survival, especially in the first few hours out of the cardiac catheterization lab. However, as he or she approaches discharge, his or her concerns change. In our experience, nurses and physicians universally report that the patient's biggest concern at discharge is, "Can I have sex?" Anticipating that customer service diagnosis and ensuring that the question is addressed is an important part of the healing process, just as the purely cardiac aspects are.

Provision of excellent customer service begins with recruitment and onboarding. Your selection process for new employees and medical staff, your orientation process, and your ongoing evaluation process must address the fact that highly trained and skilled medical and nursing staffs are better trained at and often gain more satisfaction from caring for horizontal patients with acute medical needs. They are less well trained in treating, and therefore gain less satisfaction from, more vertical customers. If they aren't getting this training in medical or nursing school—and trust us, they aren't—your organization *must* build it into the fabric of the organization.

Finally, always remember to answer the following questions:

◆ Are they patients or are they customers? *They are always both, to varying degrees.*

- Do we need clinical skills or customer service skills? *We always need both, the balance of which depends on the clinical diagnosis and the customer service diagnosis.*

Making the customer service (as well as the clinical) diagnosis and offering the right treatment is the subject of the next chapter, as we move from the "why" of healthcare customer service to the details of "how."

SURVIVAL SKILLS SUMMARY

- In every clinical encounter in your healthcare system, staff members subconsciously ask themselves, "Is this a patient, or is this a customer?"
- The more horizontal the patient is (acutely ill, dependent, less choice, less vocal), the more he is a *patient*. The more vertical (less acutely ill, independent, more choice, more vocal), the more he is a *customer*.
- The customer portion of the encounter may be considered the return we give to patients for the privilege of caring for them.
- As the patient's health improves, she increasingly becomes a customer. Thus, the patient–customer axis rotates from horizontal to vertical.
- Use the "Are they patients, or are they customers?" exercise to help your staff understand this important issue.
- Instill in your staff the constant need to ask, "Has this person's patient–customer axis rotated today?"
- Service excellence requires skills training. Almost perversely, staff think that patients (people who are very sick) have low expectations while customers (people who are in better health) have high expectations. Even though your highly productive clinicians are well trained and skilled at meeting patients' expectations, they may feel they are poorly trained in and don't enjoy meeting customers' expectations.
- Are they patients, or are they customers? *They are always both—to varying degrees—in the course of their journey through your healthcare system.*
- Service excellence is an evidence-based discipline that makes the job easier.
- It is highly unlikely that your staff has received training in this discipline. You must provide it for them and constantly and consistently reinforce it.
- Percent patient + percent customer = 100 percent.
- Treat the percent patient with technical skills and the percent customer with service excellence skills.

REFERENCE

Cushing, H. 1940. *The Life of Sir William Osler*. Hamburg, Germany: Severus Verlag.

MORE RESOURCES ON PATIENTS VERSUS CUSTOMERS

These short articles from the medical and business literature cover concepts ranging from defining patients and customers to offering strategies for change in healthcare.

Berwick, D. M. 2003. "Disseminating Innovations in Healthcare." *Journal of the American Medical Association* 289 (15): 1969–75.

Mayer, T. 2010. "Drive Service Excellence to the Next Level." *Healthcare Executive* 25 (6): 54–56.

Mayer, T. 2010. "Leadership for Great Customer Service." *Healthcare Executive* 25 (3): 66–69.

APPENDIX 3.1

Patient–CustoMeter Examples from Various Clinical Settings

Medical/Surgical Floor

Scenario 1. A patient was just transferred from the ICU, still potentially unstable, who is extremely anxious.

Scenario 2. A patient should have been discharged several days ago but is still awaiting a skilled nursing facility placement and hits his call button about ten times per hour.

Scenario 3. Same as scenario 2, but this time, the patient is your father.

Pediatrics

Scenario 1. A ten-year-old child riding his bicycle without a helmet has been struck by a car traveling 40 miles per hour. Her pulse rate is 170, her blood pressure is 70, and she is being ventilated.

Scenario 2. A three-year-old child presents to the ED at 3 o'clock in the morning, having been seen by her pediatrician at 3 o'clock in the afternoon, where a diagnosis of an ear infection was made and the patient was started on antibiotics and given fever control instructions. Now the patient has a temperature of 99.2°F (normal being 98.6°F) and the parents say they "can't get the fever down," despite the fact that no fever medication has been given and the antibiotic prescription hasn't been filled.

Scenario 3. This scenario is precisely the same as scenario 2 with one exception—this is your child or grandchild.

Intensive Care Unit

Scenario 1. A patient is admitted directly from the operating room following emergency surgery and has multiple lines and drips and is being mechanically ventilated.

Scenario 2. A patient who has no lines would have been transferred to the medical/surgical floor had a bed been available. He is constantly asking questions and hitting his call button.

Scenario 3. Same as scenario 2, except this patient is your favorite uncle.

Long-Term Care
(Note that in this example, the patient–customer axis actually changes. It is much easier to take care of the woman in scenario 1, so the staff typically call her a patient [perhaps with a bit of double entendre], while the more demented, demanding patient in scenarios 2 and 3, who has lost much of his cognitive function, is usually referred to as a patient.)

Scenario 1. A frail, 80-year-old woman "dresses for church" every morning, wondering "When will the bus to Mass be here?" but she is unfailingly kind and grateful.

Scenario 2. A man with deepening Alzheimer's disease is loud, demanding, and frequently abusive.

Scenario 3. The same as scenario 2, except this patient is your grandfather, who was always kind to you.

Part II

SURVIVAL SKILLS
FOR ACHIEVING
GREAT CUSTOMER SERVICE

Survival Skill 1: Making the Customer Service Diagnosis and Offering the Right Treatment

At this point, we move from the "why" of healthcare customer service to the "how" of implementation. In the previous chapter, we introduce the concept that every patient should receive both a clinical diagnosis (requiring technical expertise) and a customer service diagnosis (requiring service excellence skills)—and be treated for both.

Until now, most organizations have been training for technical excellence but not measuring for customer service excellence, only customer satisfaction. In fact, healthcare continues to move rapidly toward measurement of technical excellence through the Centers for Medicare & Medicaid Services' Value-Based Purchasing and Core Measures programs and an ever-increasing number of evidence-based clinical guidelines. Yet, not only is measurement of service excellence not going away but its importance and level of sophistication are increasing, to which the evolution of the HCAHPS (Hospital Consumer Assessment of Healthcare Providers and Systems) survey portion of Value-Based Purchasing attests.

Consider the following scenario, which we call "Where do I hit with the hammer?"

A man owned a car that looked great but made an awful noise when he drove it. This car made so much noise that people would point to it as it drove by and then put their fingers in their ears. The guy took it to a garage and asked the mechanic if he could fix it. The mechanic looked at the car, listened to it, and said, "I think I can help you."

The mechanic put the car on the rack with the engine running, raised it in the air, and peered up from underneath it for a minute or two. He reached over to his toolbox, pulled out a 10-pound ball peen hammer, and swung it in a broad arc, hitting the car as hard as he possibly could. Suddenly, the engine purred and the car was fixed. The mechanic brought the car down and drove it around the block, and it stayed fixed. He wrote out a bill and handed it to the customer. The bill was for $75.

The customer cried, "You charged me $75 to hit my car with a ball peen hammer?!?"

"No," the mechanic said. "I charged you 5 bucks for hitting your car with a hammer. I charged you 70 bucks for knowing *where* to hit it with the hammer."

Survival Skill 1, making the customer service diagnosis (in addition to the clinical diagnosis) and offering the right, *evidence-based* treatment for it, recognizes that we need to hit on the right clinical treatment and on the right customer service treatment. But in many hospitals and health systems, a mismatch continues to be evident between the amount of service excellence training offered and the amount needed to treat the customer service diagnosis.

WHERE ARE WE?

One of the first efforts to be undertaken in a service excellence initiative is to develop a clear sense of where you are when you start. After all, how can you know where you're going unless you know where you are? In 1994, we and our organizational colleagues began our customer service excellence journey in just that fashion, by asking patients what they thought of the customer service in our emergency department (ED). We administered questionnaires, held focus groups, conducted complaint analysis, used telephone surveys—just about any means available at the time to discover what the community thought of our customer service skills at that time. We wanted to know, *Where are we?*

What we heard from patients/customers is that our technical excellence was widely known—but expected. Although patient safety and reliability are extremely important issues in healthcare, making the right diagnosis and offering the right treatment *alone* do not suffice when it comes to how carefully and deeply patients and their families assess your services.

Adjusting the Treatment Mind-Set

Say a provider tells you she made the right diagnosis and offered the right treatment. You may want to reply, "Do you think that patient would come to our hospital if he thought he was going to get the *wrong* diagnosis and treatment?"

The fact is that technical excellence—and the stress is on *excellence*, not just competence, in today's competitive healthcare environment—is a *necessary condition* for healthcare success—it must be present for success to occur. However, it is not a *sufficient condition*. It is not enough to ensure that success occurs, and it means that the organization's *caring competence* lags its technical competence.

If you tell your staff that their caring competence is not as high as their technical competence, have you just told them that they don't care about their patients? No, of course not. However, staff members often *feel* as if you have. The point is simple. Ask yourself how much training your staff received in making the clinical diagnosis and offering the correct treatment during medical school, residency, nursing school, hospital orientation, and in-service education. Now, ask how much training they have gotten in caring competence—the customer service skills expected by your patients/customers. If your institution is like most, more than 90 percent of the training and ongoing education is geared toward technical aspects, too often to the exclusion of training in service skills. The bottom line is that you will be judged by both sets of skills, so you must train for both in a systematic and rigorous way.

MAKING THE CUSTOMER SERVICE DIAGNOSIS

The first Survival Skill involves making the customer service diagnosis *in addition to* the clinical diagnosis—not *to the exclusion of* the clinical diagnosis. Every patient needs to be fully and effectively diagnosed and treated if healthcare service success is to occur.

Your staff is probably very good at figuring out what the customer service diagnosis is—they simply haven't discussed it. To illustrate, conduct this simple exercise: Referring to the table below, show your staff a common clinical diagnosis or chief complaint (such as those listed in the left-hand column), and ask them to identify the biggest fear or concern (the customer service diagnosis) the patient or family has related to that clinical diagnosis or complaint.

Clinical Diagnosis	Fear (Customer Service Diagnosis)
Pediatric fever	"Does my child have meningitis?"
Chest pain	"Have I had a heart attack?"
Abdominal pain	"Do I have appendicitis?" "Do I have cancer?" (if the patient is 50 years of age or older)
Facial laceration	"Will I have a scar?" "Do I need to get a shot?" "Will the injury become infected?"

As you can see from the typical responses we encounter (right-hand column), the problem is not staff members' ability to figure out what the customer service diagnosis is; it is that they have never been trained to do so, much less how to treat these diagnoses. In chapters 7 through 17, which cover the various tools in our A-Team Tool Kit, we share how to encourage your leadership team to use these and other examples to help staff understand their role in diagnosing and treating customers' concerns. Next, however, we explore the two skills that contribute most to making an accurate customer service diagnosis:

◆ The ability to anticipate how the experience will play out from the customer's viewpoint
◆ The ability to create power and control options for the patient/customer

Anticipating Experiences from the Customer's Viewpoint

Rounding is one of the most important aspects of an evidence-based approach to healthcare leadership, as Quint Studer (2003) noted many years ago. We include it in the A-Team Tool Kit, and Chapter 11 discusses rounding in more detail.

For now, note that rounding provides a regular means by which to encounter customers' needs, wants, and expectations. As you and your leadership team make your rounds, seek to view healthcare not from the perspective of the individual providing it but from the perspective of the one receiving it. Patient-focused care, the Plaintree model, and the majority of the other service excellence initiatives incorporate the need to design systems and processes from the patient/customer's perspective rather than from the provider's, as has historically been done. They also operate based on the understanding that most patients and their families are confused, concerned, and often in pain when they cross your threshold. It's only logical to expect that and to anticipate their emotional as well as physical needs in advance. In turn, institutionalizing this approach makes it much easier for staff to meet those needs, fulfilling the primary goal of customer service improvement initiatives.

Further, viewing the provision-of-care experience from the patient/customer and family perspective is critical to improving patient flow at all levels of healthcare. Whether indirectly or explicitly, your organization has undoubtedly put this approach to work in efforts to improve flow. Consider the following examples:

ED
◆ Triage bypass or direct-to-room procedures
◆ Standing orders

- Bedside registration
- Physician at triage
- Fast-track programs
- Waiting areas dedicated to those awaiting test results

Inpatient units
- Be-a-bed-ahead programs
- Protocols for enabling early decision to admit
- Express admitting units
- Consistent 10:00 a.m. discharge

Outpatient services
- Outpatient cardiac catheterizations
- E-mail appointment services
- Extended hours of service

All of these approaches, and many more that have been instituted, began with the organization listening to the *voice of the customer,* which loudly proclaimed, "We want healthcare to be more responsive to our needs, more efficient, and more nimble." (These strategies are also excellent examples of improving patient flow, discussed in detail in Chapter 15.)

Simply stated, if you listen to your patients, they will tell you, even if indirectly, what their biggest fears and concerns are, forming a core part of the customer service diagnosis. (The art of effective listening is addressed in more detail in Chapter 5.)

Creating Power and Control Options for the Patient/Customer

Abraham Maslow (1998) devised his hierarchy of needs with a clear understanding that the base of that hierarchy involves the fulfillment of physiologic and psychologic safety needs—fundamental issues of power and control—in the daily lives of humans. What does this have to do with the concept of "Are they patients, or are they customers?" Find out by asking your staff this simple question:

In an encounter that is nearly 100 percent patient, what party holds primary power and control? The patient, or those providing care to the patient?

Your staff know that the more desperately ill or injured a patient is, the more he is willing to give power and control to those to whom his healthcare is entrusted.

(As emergency physicians, we can tell you with confidence that any time we have prepared to intubate patients, none of them have ever looked up and said, "By the way, where did you go to medical school?" They give the power and control to us by virtue of our presence at the bedside.)

Now consider the corollary to that question:

In an encounter that is nearly 100 percent customer,
which party holds primary power and control? The customer,
or those providing a healthcare service to the customer?

Someone who is nearly 100 percent vertical has most of the power and control in the customer–provider encounter. Your staff members don't like that balance, however, not because your staff are bad people but because they are people, and all people dislike situations in which they lack power and control, as Maslow's (1998) hierarchy implies (Exhibit 4.1).

Maslow's hierarchy of needs theory assumes that ascendance through the five discrete, yet closely related, stratifications of human needs can only occur when the needs of each lower level have been fully and completely met. More important, ascendance isn't permanent. Even if we have moved to a higher level of needs, if the needs of a lower level are suddenly not met, we descend inexorably to that lower level. Think about that possibility the next time you achieve great service

---

Exhibit 4.1: Maslow's Hierarchy of Needs

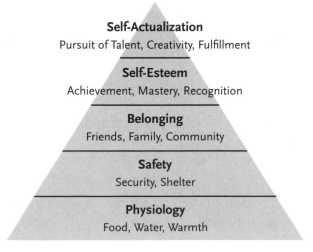

Self-Actualization
Pursuit of Talent, Creativity, Fulfillment

Self-Esteem
Achievement, Mastery, Recognition

Belonging
Friends, Family, Community

Safety
Security, Shelter

Physiology
Food, Water, Warmth

---

scores (experiencing the fulfillment of self-esteem and perhaps self-actualization) and then learn shortly after that your nursing areas are consistently and persistently short-staffed (a threat to physiological and safety needs). That sound you hear is the organization sliding down the side of the pyramid, and the organization's morale and service scores will quickly follow.

Coming back to the power/control dynamic, the more horizontal someone is, the more she *is willing to give up* power and control; the more vertical, the more she *insists on holding* power and control. Patients are fighting for the vertical, trying not just to get better but also to regain power and control over their lives. Staff must understand this dynamic and work with the patient as the patient–customer axis shifts during the course of the patient's journey through the healthcare system. Offering the patient power and control options works for both parties. Examples of such options, and the benefits they achieve, abound in healthcare and include the following:

- Better results are seen when prostate cancer patients assist in the decision whether surgery or radiation is the best treatment for them.
- Medication compliance improves, and fewer side effects occur, when patients are allowed to participate in choosing among medications with similar efficacy.
- Better compliance and earlier resolution of symptoms are seen when patients, or their parents if the ill person is a child, have a choice in which antibiotic therapy to undergo.
- Patients who are given the opportunity to select from a list of dietary options, or even to choose the time they eat, adhere more completely to nutrition guidelines.
- Shorter inpatient stays are seen when patients are kept informed of their progress toward discharge during their stay.

As indicated by the last bullet point above, one of the most significant sources of power in healthcare is information. Teach your staff to share information (power) actively, aggressively, even audaciously. For example, we advise the use of COWS— not the animals but rather **c**omputers **o**n **w**heels—in healthcare. Put electrons to work to give patients information, and therefore power, by sharing information electronically at the bedside about the patient's care, especially laboratory and imaging studies. Many people learn better with visual imagery representing the information than by simply listening to a description of it.

EXPECTATION CREATION

Let your patients know what to expect. The more their expectations are managed, the more they feel some control over their situation and the happier they tend to be. You've seen previews in the movie theater—use that concept with your patients to give them a sense of what's to come.

The Expectation Creation Concept as Practiced by Disney

Not only does expectation creation let the patient/customer know what to expect but it also matches that information with a reasonably specific time frame. The Walt Disney Company is a master of the art and science of expectation creation. Take, for example, the waiting line for a ride at a Disney theme park. A sign is posted at the beginning of the line for many popular rides that says, "Wait from here is 40 minutes." The sign presents the customer with a couple of options: She can decide that 40 minutes is too long to wait and move on to the next attraction, perhaps returning later when the line may be shorter. Or the ride-goer can join the line and check her watch so she knows how close she is to entering the ride. Disney then sets about turning her this way and that as she proceeds through the line. Often, video monitors are positioned at strategically located spots to show previews of the ride or to provide a change of scenery to make the time pass more quickly—all designed to keep the rider informed, mark her progress, and make the wait easier. The folks at Disney know that *it's not how much time the customer spends, it's how she spends the time.*

Exceeding Expectations

Finally, it's that customer's turn, and she's on the ride. She glances at her watch and realizes, "It's only been 34 minutes. Great!" She might even think, "We got in faster than 40 minutes—we must have received the VIP treatment!"

The Disney experts in expectation creation told us they actually expect that 92 percent of ride-goers will be on the ride within 32 minutes of the time they pass the 40-minute mark sign. They create an expectation that they intend to not only meet but exceed.

What does this example have to do with healthcare? Next time you are on administrative rounds, ask one of the inpatients, "What's going to happen to you today? What's on the agenda? Where are you in your journey back to health?" The vast majority of the patients in your hospital have no clue—not because they are less than intelligent and curious, but because you are not using *expectation creation* to let them know where they are and what to expect. And that means, unlike the 92 percent of Disney theme park customers who wait in line and have their expectations exceeded, most of your patients are poised for a letdown in customer service.

How, then, do you exceed expectations? As at Disney, your staff can reasonably estimate how long a process should take. With that information, they can give the patient a time estimate that exceeds the typical time frame. For example, if the member of your staff attending to a patient who is awaiting a chest X-ray believes that the procedure will take about 45 minutes to complete under normal conditions, he should tell the patient, "I believe the chest X-ray will take an hour to an hour and 15 minutes. But I'll see if I can move it along faster for you." When the chest film is completed after only 45 minutes (or even 55 minutes), the patient has reason to be pleased with the service provided.

Expectation creation through the sharing of information has given this patient a sense of power and control. Every patient who crosses your threshold should experience nothing less, so expectation creation is a skill at which everyone in healthcare needs to be adept.

More About Communicating Expectations

Teaching staff to reliably inform patients and families through the use of specific skills is an important first step in offering the right, evidence-based treatment for their customer service diagnosis. We present the process for communicating reasonable expectations in Exhibit 4.2 and discuss each step in detail in the following paragraphs, with some comparisons to B-Team behavior.

Exhibit 4.2: Treating the Customer Service Diagnosis: Managing Expectations

1. Introduce yourself in a disciplined, professional fashion (consider applying the AIDET formula).
2. Address family members and bring them into the clinical encounter, as guided by the patient.
3. Provide information as soon as it becomes available.
4. Establish a high level of professionalism—you are always onstage.
5. Check the patient's progress multiple times.
6. Never underestimate the value of creature comforts and dignity enhancers, such as pillows, warm blankets, water and food when desired (as medically appropriate), and timely information.

Introduce Yourself

Every leader and manager has received complaints in which the patient said, "People were coming into my room and they didn't even tell me who they were!" Our natural reaction is, "No way that could have happened—we teach our staff to introduce themselves."

The problem is a simple human one, as we've noted previously: When we (staff members) are ready to talk, they (patients/customers) are not ready to listen. Many aspects of the hospital experience distract patients, including their fears about their disease or injury and their presence in an unfamiliar environment. And the fact is, we usually *do* walk into their rooms unannounced. So it is not surprising that patients aren't completely focused when we introduce ourselves. For all these reasons, it is important to have a reliable and systematic way for staff to do so. Our approach is to make a habit of saying simply,

> "Good morning, Mrs. Jones. I am Dr. Mayer, and I am the emergency physician who will be taking care of you today."

The communication seems direct and uncomplicated, but it contains a great deal of important information:

1. Good morning (pleasant salutation), Mrs. Jones (using the patient's name).
2. I (personal pronoun) am Dr. Mayer (an identifiable person with a clear title),
3. and I am the emergency physician (a clear statement of the role played)
4. who will be taking care of (expression of care, not some impersonal relationship)
5. you (the patient—very important) today.

All language has meaning, and all behavior has meaning. All great speakers have learned that the first minute of their speeches must be clearly presented, well rehearsed, and straightforward in meaning. Nothing about that first minute should be left up to chance, and rehearsing the speech verbatim is the only way to avoid unintended misunderstandings. (See the Oscar-winning movie *The King's Speech* for a wonderfully lyrical example of this.)

So, if you wouldn't leave a speech to chance, why would you leave your initial interaction with someone with whom you will be sharing intimate knowledge about his healthcare—who also is a stranger—to chance? Clearly, you shouldn't. The language used to communicate with the patient when you first walk into his room is extremely powerful and sets the tone for the remainder of the experience.

B-Team members are convinced they are communicating appropriately, even correctly, when in fact their introductions lack much important information:

"Hello, I'm your doctor. Why are you here?"

"I'm your nurse. You don't need anything, do you?"

"I'm here to take you to X-ray."

To B-Team members, these "introductions" sound fine. But they usually are not adequate communications. "Fine" is not what you want to experience when you are a patient, and it is definitely not enough to satisfy your family. One effective way to ensure that the healthcare team's messages—including introductions—are communicated accurately is to mark information on a whiteboard in each patient's room.

The Studer Group (Studer 2003) uses the acronym AIDET to help organizations standardize introductions:

Acknowledge the patient and family.
Introduce yourself and what your role on the team is.
Indicate **d**uration—how long the process will likely take (a form of expectation creation).
Explain what will happen in simple, straightforward terms.
Thank them for choosing your hospital and for the privilege of caring for them.

Address Family Members and Make Them a Part of the Clinical Encounter

Embracing the role of the family in the healing process, in which the goal is to move patients from horizontal to vertical, is another example of a best practice that is generally well known but often poorly executed. We all know that family involvement is critical to healing, but have we treated it as such, systematically and in an evidence-based fashion? Probably not.

Here's an example of how not to proceed in such an exchange with family:

An ED doctor walks into the room of a young woman with abdominal pain and sees an "older man" at the bedside. The doctor smiles, extends his hand, and says, "Hello, I am Dr. Cates, the emergency physician, and I will be taking care of your daughter today."

"I beg your pardon," he says. "That is my wife you're referring to."

You then say, incredulously, "That's your *wife?*"

(Trust us, we've all been there.)

The point is, your staff should be taught in orientation and through ongoing education sessions to make *sure* they know who they are talking to. A better way to handle the above situation is to follow these steps:

1. Address the patient first.
    Example: "Hi, I'm Dr. Loya, and I am the hospital medicine specialist—your doctor. I'm taking care of you today and will be coordinating your care during your stay."
2. Extend a warm greeting to the person in the room with the patient.
    Example: "Hi, I'm Dr. Loya . . ."
3. Establish who that person is and what his or her relationship to the patient is.
    Example: ". . . and you are—?"
4. Acknowledge their relationship in a warm and welcoming way.
    Example: "Family and friends are an important part of the healing process."
5. Keep the patient fully and completely in control of what information should—and should not—be shared with the family member during the course of care.
    Example: "I'll need to perform a physical examination now. Would you prefer that I do that privately?" If the patient's answer is yes, ask the family or friends, "Would you please wait outside while we complete the examination?"
6. Respect the patient's wishes at all times. Once the family is outside of the room, it is appropriate to confirm those wishes with the patient. Sensitive information is often elicited from the patient when he is in the privacy of the patient–caregiver relationship.
    Example: "Please let us know if you would like us to share the results of your care with you alone first or if you would like your family informed at the same time. Your privacy is very important to us."
7. Ensure that those personal patient preferences are respected by communicating them to the other members of the team, both verbally and on the patient's health record.
    Example: "I've just spoken to Mrs. Thompson, and she prefers that we discuss any and all test results with her, and she will decide when and how to share those results with her family."

Provide Information as Soon as It Becomes Available

We've said it before, and we all know it is true: Information is power. And the more acutely ill or injured the patient, the more powerful that information is. In

Chapter 3, we note that every patient with chest pain thinks she is having a heart attack, every patient with abdominal pain thinks he has appendicitis or cancer, and every parent of a child with fever worries that the child has meningitis. The anxiety of anticipating the worst outcome is not healthy and should not be prolonged more than necessary. As soon as we have information that proves the patient is not suffering the worst-case illness, we should let the patient know.

Following are some examples for relating this type of news:

"While you do have chest pain, your EKG looks completely normal, your chest X-ray is clear, and it doesn't look like this is a heart attack."

"Great news! The abdominal CT scan we performed is normal, and I don't see any evidence of appendicitis (or cancer)."

"It can be scary when your child has a high fever, but his physical exam is completely normal. Most importantly, I wouldn't be able to bend his neck like this if he had meningitis."

We discuss the role of scripts as examples of evidence-based language—which serves to make our jobs easier—in more detail in Chapter 12.

Of course, there is more to communicating information than sharing it in a timely way. Follow these simple rules to ensure that you're exceeding the patient's expectations and respecting her need to retain some power and control:

1. *Tell the patient why the test is being performed.* Every lab test or imaging study has a purpose—to confirm (or, more often, rule out) a potential diagnosis or disease.
2. *Tell the patient how long the test is expected to take.* (See the section titled "Expectation Creation" and the concept of previews, discussed earlier.)
3. *Let the patient know you will give her the results as rapidly as possible.* In Chapter 1, we mention T. S. Eliot's wisdom about the "shadow" between the idea and the action. Make the shadow as short as possible.
4. *The more potentially acute and life threatening the results of the test, the faster the results should be delivered.*

Let's apply these steps to a common example. Say a 65-year-old man with an 80-pack-per-year history of smoking arrives at the hospital after three weeks of coughing and producing greenish-yellow sputum. The healthcare providers cannot help thinking, "Why in the world did he *wait* so long to come in?" The answer is simple and universal: He knows what the worst news could be, and he had hoped the symptoms would go away. His thinking represents the customer service diagnosis we discuss in detail in the previous chapter.

Everyone—and we mean *everyone,* from the patient to the family to the nurses to the doctor—knows the worst fear is of lung cancer. The healthcare providers ask themselves, "What test do we conduct to make the diagnosis?"

In this case, the answer is the chest radiograph. Next, the providers consider how long it should take from the time the chest X-ray is taken until they are in the room giving the patient the test results.

The answer for the patient and family is, "extremely fast," and that is the only answer that matters. Otherwise, the patient and the family are left to wonder if the patient will live or face an untimely death, with no sense of how long they must agonize waiting for the results.

We need to do a better job in healthcare of getting information to the patient as soon as it becomes available. Every time a patient has a CT scan of the abdomen in the morning, waits all day wondering if she has appendicitis or cancer, and then hears, "Your doctor will give you your results in the morning," we have failed.

Establish and Maintain a High Level of Professionalism

When visiting Walt Disney World to study the theme park's approach to customer service and reliability, we learned about the concept of "onstage–offstage." Disney prides itself on hiring "cast members" rather than employees, each of whom plays a role in the experience created for Disney's guests. That experience is expected to be reliably and predictably pleasant, even exciting, because every cast member understands his or her onstage role.

For Disney, *onstage* means whenever and wherever the cast members are seen, heard, or observed. *Offstage* constitutes an entire city below the surface and behind the fences of Disney where the cast members are not required to stay in character and can take a break from their "performances."

In healthcare, however, there is no offstage. We are always in front of the patients and their families. In the clinical areas, whether providing service in patients' rooms, walking down the hallways, or sitting in the nurses' station, we are very much onstage in that there are always people watching us, measuring our professionalism, taking our mien, observing how we behave and interact. Here's a simple truth about maintaining professionalism in healthcare:

All of us are always onstage. The healthcare professions truly are performance art.

What about when we are on break, at lunch, or even walking into or out of the hospital? Aren't we offstage then? Hardly. We are observed by many others even in these simple movements. And because those "others" are patients, families, and visitors, we are wise to remember that it is precisely when patients or families get most angry and "in your face" that we need to be most calm, professional, and compassionate (see Chapter 9 for a discussion on B-Team patients).

We tend to think of always being watched as problematic because we might "get caught." But think of all the folks who have gotten caught doing something great. Staff get a tremendous boost when they are acknowledged for being professional, as the following feedback example demonstrates:

> "I was a family member visiting on 9 West and observed one of the most obnoxious patients, who was literally yelling at and berating the staff. But your nurse/doctor/tech/housekeeper was so calm and professional that he completely defused the situation. I just wanted to compliment him for his consummate professionalism."

Make sure your staff know they are *always* onstage, and coach them on how to take advantage of that position. As we discuss in more detail in Chapter 12, providing healthcare service is a form of "performance art."

Check Patients' Progress Multiple Times

Given the limited amount of time available to be spent with a patient over the course of a clinical encounter, patients and families prefer to have that exposure broken up into discrete, information-filled, brief encounters rather than one long encounter.

For example, during an ED patient visit, the emergency physician might spend a total of 15 to 20 minutes in the room. Does that patient prefer that the doctor spend 12 to 15 minutes of that time in the initial encounter and then offer a brief summary that takes several minutes at discharge or spend 10 minutes up front and then check back with the patient several times of briefer duration? Almost without exception, patients prefer the multiple-visit encounter; they report higher satisfaction for having been kept informed (Mayer et al. 2014).

We have learned to step to the door/curtain while walking past a patient's room on the way to see another patient and ask, "Is that pain medication helping?" Or, "Have they taken your X-ray? Great, I'll check the result after I see this next patient." Or, "Have you thought of any questions I can answer for you?"

Create an Environment Replete with Creature Comforts and Dignity Enhancers

Never forget the power of water, juice, and warm blankets in the healthcare experience. Are we curing dehydration, hypoglycemia, or hypothermia with these thoughtful gestures? Of course not. But we are showing that we care and notice individuals in what is, to be frank, a highly depersonalizing environment. Think about what we do with patients in the healthcare system:

1. Give them a number.
2. Have them strip and put on a revealing and uncomfortable gown, which can be maddeningly difficult to secure.
3. Assign them a priority level (triage or level of acuity).
4. Remove all semblance of power and control.
5. Put them in a cold, unwelcoming environment. (We talk about how nice our patient rooms are, but seriously, would you decorate your house that way?)
6. Keep them waiting in the midst of the most troubling anxiety they may have ever encountered.

When you put it that way, they sound more like incarcerates than patients—and that is precisely the way they feel.

In the midst of an environment that seems to have been carefully designed to strip patients of their sense of dignity and self-worth, offering the simple gestures that consider their most basic needs has tremendous impact. We were fortunate to have learned early in our careers not only to be observant of our surroundings from the patient and family perspective but also to answer the needs we identify. Both of us have heard nurses and other healthcare workers say, "There goes Dr. Cates/Mayer with his 'dignity enhancers'!"

So what exactly are dignity enhancers? Dignity enhancers are the simple efforts we all can take to ensure that we are respecting the dignity of our patients in the often dehumanizing environment of healthcare. Collectively, they are a positive and proactive effort to consider how we would want to be treated if we were the patient.

Who should provide those dignity enhancers and creature comforts? Whoever observes the need for them. From long experience as emergency physicians practicing in one of the highest-volume and highest-acuity EDs in the United States, we can tell you it is faster, easier, and more practical for us to retrieve a warm blanket for our patients than it is to find an ED technologist to do it for us. The techs are busy, our time is well spent on the task, and the reaction of the patient and family is gratifying beyond belief.

VERBAL SKILLS AND COMPLAINT/COMPLIMENT ANALYSIS

Many of the best examples of making the customer service diagnosis and offering the right treatment involve a combination of verbal skills and simple courtesies. Examples include those listed in Exhibit 4.3.

As your customer service initiative grows and gains momentum, your staff will recognize and develop more and more of these verbal skills. They are nothing more (or less) than A-Team behaviors, all of which work by making your job easier—no matter who "you" are. These verbal A-Team behaviors should be analyzed and discussed at every staff meeting to engender group—not individual—learning.

| Patient compliment | What were the A-Team behaviors that generated the compliment? | Celebrate, accentuate, and circulate them. |
| Patient complaint | What were the B-Team behaviors that generated the complaint? | Identify, isolate, and eliminate them. |

Although complaint and compliment analysis and instant feedback to the staff are essential, they are probably the most neglected concepts in service excellence. As we discuss in the next chapter, service recovery is crucial. Through service recovery,

Exhibit 4.3: Examples of Diagnosing and Treating Healthcare Situations Using Verbal Skills

Situation	Verbal Skill
Patient/family looks lost in hallway	"May I help you find where you're going? It can be a bit confusing around here."
Elevator etiquette	"After you, please." No discussions of patient care or sensitive information on elevators. "Let me move over to make room for you."
Child with laceration in ED triage	"You've come to the right place; we take care of these all the time."
Patient checking in for elective procedure	"Welcome, Mr. Smith, we've been expecting you."
All patients	"Thank you for choosing our hospital and trusting us with your care."

not only do we hear the voice of the customer but also we have a chance to give that feedback instantly to our staff.

SURVIVAL SKILLS SUMMARY

- Patients and their families are widely aware of our technical excellence—but this excellence is *expected*.
- Our caring competence—our customer service skills—is generally not as highly rated as our technical skills. Most healthcare delivery in the United States is much more heavily geared toward technical skills, with much less emphasis on service skills. Without neglecting the former, find a way to place considerably more emphasis on training for customer service, both in orientation and in ongoing education.
- Just as every patient has a technical, clinical diagnosis, he or she also has a customer service diagnosis.
- Survival Skill 1 is to make the customer service diagnosis and offer the right treatment.
- Anticipate experiences from the customer's viewpoint, and change your systems to reflect this customer focus.
  - Incorporate the voice of the customer into process redesign by hardwiring efficient and effective patient flow throughout the system.
- Help your staff learn to create power and control options for both patients and customers.
- Use the insights of Maslow's hierarchy of needs in the power–control equation.
- Expectation creation is a powerful tool—put it to work.
  - Have the staff introduce themselves in a consistent, disciplined fashion.
  - Address family members and make them a part of the clinical encounter.
  - Provide information as soon as possible.
  - Remember that you are always onstage.
  - Check on the patient's progress multiple times.
  - Deliver creature comforts and dignity enhancers.
- Use compliment analysis (A-Team behaviors) and complaint analysis (B-Team behaviors) to identify verbal skills that produce service excellence.
- Develop and use scripts to accentuate A-Team behaviors.

REFERENCES

Maslow, A. H. 1998. *Maslow on Management.* New York: Wiley.

Mayer, T. A., J. Kaplan, R. W. Strauss, and R. J. Cates. 2014. "Customer Service in Emergency Medicine." In *Strauss and Mayer's Emergency Department Management,* edited by R. W. Strauss and T. A. Mayer. New York: McGraw-Hill.

Studer, Q. 2003. *Hardwiring Excellence: Purpose, Worthwhile Work, Making a Difference.* Gulf Breeze, FL: Fire Starter Press.

MORE RESOURCES ON MAKING THE CUSTOMER SERVICE DIAGNOSIS

Berry, L. L., and N. Bendapudi. 2003. "Clueing in Customers." *Harvard Business Review* 81 (2): 100–106.

Berry, L. L., and K. D. Seltman. 2008. *Leadership Lessons from Mayo Clinic: Inside One of the World's Most Respected Service Organizations.* New York: McGraw-Hill.

Service from the customer's perspective at the Mayo Clinic, as seen through the eyes of a legend in service writings.

CHAPTER 5

Survival Skill 2: Negotiating Agreement on, and Resolution of, Expectations

As a healthcare leader, how often do you negotiate? Every day, twice a day, four times a day, all day? It depends, of course, but few would argue that negotiation is an essential competency for leaders and managers as well as for bedside providers of healthcare. Of course, you negotiate contracts, payment rates, issues between departments, and other areas of a legal nature, but we are referring to something more fundamental and far more frequent in healthcare. Throughout your organization, negotiations regarding patient care are occurring daily, hourly, even by the minute. Consider the following statements—don't they all involve negotiation?

Charge nurse to staff nurses: "I need someone to take this patient."

Shift supervisor to registration bed board: "The emergency department needs three critical care beds ASAP."

Emergency physician to emergency department (ED) charge nurse: "We are two nurses down and have ten boarders—how should we pull the team together to give the best patient care we can in these circumstances?"

Operating suite supervisor to CEO: "Dr. Smith wants more block operating room time, or he says he'll take his business elsewhere."

Chief of medicine to director of radiology: "Why can't we get the radiology reports on the chart (or the computer) before 8:00 a.m. when the doctors round on their patients?"

CEO to department director: "Our institution has committed to service excellence throughout the organization. I've noticed that your unit's customer service scores have been trending downward. I've asked my assistant to block a couple of hours so we can discuss this in some depth. For part of that time, I've asked Jane Smith to join us, since her unit has had great scores, so she can share some ideas that could be of help."

Emergency physician to patient's family: "I know you feel your mother needs to be admitted to the hospital, but her illness is not one that usually meets the criteria that we think of for admission. Why don't I discuss it with her physician so he can make a final decision?"

Cardiologist to emergency physician: "Can you talk to the hospitalist and have her admit this patient to the chest pain unit, and I will consult?"

All of these scenarios involve negotiations among members of the healthcare team. An even more common negotiation occurs thousands of times a day in every healthcare system in the United States, whether in the ED, inpatient units, outpatient settings, or long-term care facilities: the negotiation between patients/customers and caregivers about their expectations for healthcare.

As we discuss in Chapter 2, the patient has one set of expectations, and those who work in healthcare often have another. Without training in negotiation skills, how can we hope to resolve these differences and align expectations? This chapter addresses the second Survival Skill, negotiating agreement on, and resolution of, expectations.

The unfortunate fact is that the majority of healthcare providers—particularly clinicians—have never taken a formal course on negotiation. Ask yourself these questions: Does *your* hospital or healthcare system, as a part of its routine orientation, offer material on how to negotiate? Is negotiation addressed in your management team meetings, your in-service educational programs, and your continuing medical education offerings for your physicians? We're guessing the answer for most of you is "No." Our view is that while many of us have tacitly received at least the most rudimentary didactic training in this essential skill, very few healthcare systems explicitly train their staff in basic negotiation skills.

WHAT IS NEGOTIATION?

While there are many definitions of *negotiation*, perhaps the simplest and most pragmatic is this:

> *Negotiation is an interactive process between two or more people designed to achieve a desired outcome through effective communication.*

At the outset, negotiation is a *people process* that requires excellent communication skills, about which we say much more later. For the moment, keep this simple syllogism in mind:

The best **negotiators** are the best **learners.**
The best **learners** are the best **listeners.**
Therefore, the best **negotiators** are the best **listeners.**

THE ROLE OF LISTENING IN NEGOTIATION

Literally hundreds of books have been published on the topic of listening (we have listed a number of excellent resources at the end of this chapter), which speaks to the fact that the art of listening is not a passive, easy thing but is one subject to teaching. As an example of the depth of the listening problem in healthcare, both our research (Mayer et al. 2014) and that of Dr. Jerome Groopman (2007) indicate that when interviewing patients, physicians take an average of . . . 18 seconds to interrupt the patient! That is truly stunning—18 seconds is a very, very short time in which a patient is allowed to tell his story before the average physician interrupts. Our research also indicates that nurses interrupt patients within 54 seconds of initiating a discussion with them (a fact my neonatal ICU nurse–wife points out indicates that nurses are at least three times better than doctors at listening) (Mayer et al. 2014).

How to Improve Our Listening Skills

All of us in healthcare need to become better listeners. Here are a few ideas on how we do that.

First, we need to be *ready* to listen—prepared to have our ears open and our mouths closed—so the patient can tell his story. Part of this preparation can be guided by the important work of psychologist Albert Mehrabian (1981), who showed that verbal content is but one small component of a message:

Components of Effective Persuasion	Percentage of Message
Verbal content	7
Vocal expression	38
Visual cues	55

We've all had the experience of listening to people and finding that the words and the music don't match, in that they say one thing with their words while the broader picture, as conveyed by body language and tone of voice, is much more complicated. Examples include the following:

- A patient stands with arms crossed and teeth clenched and says in a loud voice, "I'm not angry!"
- The parent of a critically ill child, visibly shaking and with tears in her eyes, says, "I'm fine—really, I'm fine, don't worry about me."
- A physician with a long history of angry and inappropriate behavior says in a flat monotone, "Oh, yes, I really enjoy these sensitivity training sessions."

In each case, the words themselves say one thing but convey only about 7 percent of the message. Good listening is a key to successful negotiations and requires taking into account the entire package of the communication.

Second, we should regularly practice one of the most useful techniques to improve listening: *active listening*. It is so important that we discuss it in more detail in Chapter 7, but for the moment, we note that active listening helps (1) assure the patient and family that we are actively engaged in the conversation and (2) ensure that the patient's history is accurate, that we have a shared understanding of the clinical workup, that she knows where she is in the healthcare journey from horizontal to vertical, and that she is aware of what will occur in the course of care delivery.

Active listening has been defined in many ways. Here is our definition:

Active listening is a communication tool in which the listener systematically feeds back what she has heard the speaker say in order to

- *improve clarity of the message,*
- *make listening a participative process, and*
- *ensure common ground is gained in the ongoing process of communication.*

Third, it is essential for healthcare providers to make sure that the patient clearly understands the stated *desired outcome*. In other words, success should be defined before you enter into negotiations about the patient's care so you know what it looks like when you achieve it. All too frequently, the people involved in negotiations *assume* the desired outcome is clear, mutual, and shared, yet each party has its discrete definition of what that outcome is.

Stephen Covey (2013), in his book *The 7 Habits of Highly Effective People,* notes as his second habit to "begin with the end in mind." Unless we start with a clear and mutual definition of a successful outcome, we shouldn't be surprised if we end up in a different place than we thought or hoped we would.

Always enter into negotiations with as clear a definition of success as possible, understanding that any interaction among people will result in a refined definition over time.

Of course, defining success is not the same as having rigid, preconceived notions of precisely how the end will be achieved. But it does take into account the considerable experience of healthcare leaders, managers, and clinicians to anticipate, to the extent possible, how success might be framed.

Negotiating the effective resolution of patients' expectations requires us to think in advance of some possible end results. For example, a patient with prostate cancer might be given several options with regard to his treatment. What those options are and how they are presented should certainly be important sources of preparation for the conversation. Similarly, an emergency physician seeing a young athlete with a concussion, along with her parents, needs to be prepared to discuss the most effective diagnostic and treatment options, perhaps in the following manner:

"Mr. and Mrs. Lopez, the history of your daughter's head injury today, as well as the complete physical and neurological exam I have done, makes it very clear that she has suffered a concussion. A concussion is a form of brain trauma that is relatively mild to moderate in nature but that doesn't require CT scanning of the head to diagnose. In fact, detailed study of concussions has shown that CT scans of the head produce an unnecessary radiation risk and don't add in any way to making the diagnosis or deciding the right treatment.

"Most athletes recover from their concussions over a period of days, after a time of physical and mental rest designed to let the brain heal at its fastest pace. This sheet summarizes the gradual return-to-participation protocol, which is based on the best evidence available, including cognitive rest—so no computers or video games for the next several days. I will discuss this in more detail with your doctor and give her a copy of this protocol. Mom, Dad, Janna, do you have any questions?"

This is a simple example that shows the importance of defining success prior to the negotiation by preparing. Of particular significance is calling on evidence-based clinical guidelines whenever possible to help the patient and family make diagnostic and treatment decisions. In the case of a young athlete with a concussion, parents often come to the ED expecting their child to undergo a CT scan. As we discuss in Chapter 2 and reemphasize later, it is critical to discover such expectations at the outset of the clinical encounter. When there are discrepancies between their expectation (a CT scan of the head) and our expectations (CT scan is not needed and poses radiation risks), relying on evidence-based guidelines can be very helpful in the negotiating process.

APPROACHES TO SUCCESSFUL NEGOTIATING

With all these thoughts about listening and communication in mind, let's turn to the skill of negotiation itself. In our view, the finest book on negotiation is the simple yet nuanced text by Fisher, Ury, and Patton (1991), *Getting to Yes*. (Based on their experience with the Harvard Negotiation Project, the book is filled with insights and delineates the quintessential approach to successful negotiation.)

They list four key principles in their approach to successful negotiation:

1. Separate the people from the problem.
2. Focus on interests and principles, not on positions.
3. Invent options for mutual gain.
4. Insist on prospective, objective criteria by which to define success.

Separate the People from the Problem

In negotiating agreement and resolution with our patients, the principle of keeping the people separate from the problem is paramount. The quote by Sir William Osler (mentioned on page 39) that "It is much more important to know what sort of a patient has a disease than what sort of a disease a patient has," reflects this principle.

At BestPractices, as an example to all of our clinicians, we strive to always remember to put the patient first, a sentiment that is supported by the 3 Rules of our mission statement:

1. **Always** do the right thing for the patient.
2. Do the right thing for those who take care of the patient.
3. Don't confuse Rule 1 and Rule 2.

The Mayo Clinic does the same with its motto "Patient first," as Berry and Seltman (2008) point out in their excellent book, *Leadership Lessons from Mayo Clinic.* Keeping the focus constantly on the patient first in healthcare is an excellent first step toward ensuring that we separate the people from the problem.

Focus on Interests and Principles, Not on Positions

A relatively recent development in healthcare delivery serves as an example of the second principle, focusing on interests, not positions, and is seen every day in our hospitals and healthcare systems. With the growing availability of healthcare information, patients often come to their clinical encounter armed with expectations based on pages of research they have conducted on the Internet. In some cases, our clinicians may respond huffily, "Wait a moment, I'm the doctor (or nurse), and I'll be making the decisions here!" Such a response demonstrates a focus on positions instead of principles and interests. In the information age—and we are decidedly in the information age—the following maxim should be helpful for your staff:

The speed of expectations is the speed of information, which is the speed of electrons.

It is no longer uncommon for patients and their families to access information on the Internet about their clinical problem, and the diagnostic and therapeutic implications thereof, from their smartphone *during the course of their care.* So always keep in mind that patients' expectations could actually increase during the encounter. Here's an example:

Hospitalist to inpatient: "Today we are going to get a repeat chest X-ray."

Inpatient: "I've been reading on the Internet that the amount of radiation from repeated chest X-rays may put me at risk for developing cancer. Do I really need to have the X-ray done?"

Hospitalist: "Excellent question. In your case, we do need the chest X-ray because there has been a change in your clinical status."

Invent Options for Mutual Gain

Perhaps the most important aspect of negotiation discussed in *Getting to Yes* is the third principle—the concept of inventing options for mutual gain (Fisher, Ury, and Patton 1991). Many people define negotiation as "win-win" or "meeting in the middle"—or, more simply, "compromise." While these definitions sound workable, how do they apply in action? Consider the following interchange.

Nursing supervisor: "I need you to take this patient—the ED is getting slammed!"

Medical/surgical floor charge nurse: "We can't. We just took two patients four hours ago."

Nursing supervisor: "Okay . . . how about taking half of a patient?"

In this situation, meeting in the middle, meeting halfway, or compromising doesn't seem to work. What we need to do is to *invent options for mutual gain*—particularly the patient's gain. Now let's revisit the negotiation. The parentheses are used to emphasize the power of carefully selected negotiation language and obviously would not be a part of what is actually said.

Nursing supervisor to medical/surgical nurse: "Julie (using people's names is powerful), I need your help with a critical issue we have (enlisting help versus giving orders, defining the importance, and using the plural pronoun). The ED is getting slammed (a fact); every unit, including yours, has been getting patients all day (more facts). I need you and three other units each to take a patient (we're all sharing a heavy load). If we can get these four patients out of the ED, we can avoid rerouting them or shutting off the operating rooms" (the consequences if we can't work this out, with the stress on *we*, not *me* or *you*).

Med/surg nurse: "Well, we're getting slammed too (a fact), but we'll do our part. Can you give us a breather after this patient?"

Nursing supervisor: "Absolutely (positive feedback), as long as it doesn't get any worse and we aren't putting patients at risk" (conditional affirmation with the patient coming first).

Conversations like these are negotiations, occurring hundreds of times a day in your organization, so as a leader, your decision whether to invest in negotiation skills training for your staff is extremely important. Negotiation involves three simple steps, each of which is discussed later in the "Negotiation Steps" section:

1. Discover your expectations.
2. Discover their expectations.
3. Invent options for mutual gain.

Insist on Prospective, Objective Criteria

The fourth principle, insisting on prospective, objective criteria by which to define success, is simply another way of defining success through a desired outcome, as we discuss earlier, but it is an essential principle in every aspect of healthcare. We work in an environment in which metrics-based management is the foundation of all of our strategic plans and, in almost every institution, a central element by which our performance plans are rewarded. One of the founding principles of our physician group, BestPractices, and our parent corporations, EmCare and Envision Healthcare Services, is "Delivering the results that matter to our patients and our partners." As we navigate the perpetual whitewater of change in which we find ourselves in healthcare, at least we have the steady beacon of established metrics with which we can view our progress.

The same principle of objective criteria applies in healthcare negotiations. Consider the examples that follow.

Boarders in the Emergency Department

ED charge nurse to nursing supervisor: "We are up to six boarders [patients admitted to the hospital but who have not been assigned a bed yet] who have been waiting more than two hours for beds, and patients are still coming through the door at a steady rate. I need beds, and I need them now!"

Nursing supervisor: "I can get you four beds, but it might take a while. You know we're coming up on change of shift."

ED charge nurse: "Define 'a while.'"

Nursing supervisor: "Probably at least four hours."

ED charge nurse: "Let me ask you a question. If these boarders were *your* mom or dad, would four *more* hours on an ED stretcher be OK?"

Nursing supervisor (after a pause): "I guess not."

ED charge nurse: "How about this? Give me two beds within an hour, two more beds within two hours, and the last two beds within four hours. I'll work with the ED charge doc to prioritize them, and I'll use our techs to transport them."

Nursing supervisor: "OK. I'll let the charge nurses on the floor know to expedite discharges, and I'll approve the overtime for housekeeping to stay and clean the beds as fast as possible."

ED charge nurse: "Great. Once you've alerted the charge nurses on the floors, come down here, and you and I can round on the boarders, tell them the plan, and let them 'put a face to the name' of the people who are responsible."

This is the type of problem that many hospitals deal with every day. Here, the example uses objective criteria by specifying the number of beds, the time frame, and the processes by which the outcome will be obtained. (It also builds in the concept of rounding.)

Poor Operating Room (OR) Utilization

Here's another example of using objective criteria in negotiation:

Chief operating officer (COO) to chairman of Anesthesia: "I really need your help. We are running at horrific OR rates. We are at only 50 percent effective capacity, despite a full slate of scheduled cases. Any idea what's going on?"

Anesthesia chair: "We've been watching this very closely, and we've found that the outpatient surgeries are killing us. Most of those patients haven't had a pre-op clearance. They get to the day of surgery and we find out they need lab or X-ray prior to surgery, so the case gets postponed or canceled."

COO: "Are you saying we can get rid of the majority of our OR utilization problem by ensuring that outpatient surgery patients have appropriate preoperative clearance?"

Anesthesia chair: "Absolutely. And we can fix it by holding a 'preoperative clinic,' whose sole function is to evaluate these patients ahead of surgery to make sure they are medically clear for their procedure."

COO: "What do we need to do to fix this?"

Anesthesia chair: "We need a place to see them, someone to schedule them, and someone to do the evaluations. We've looked into this, and we can use two currently unused rooms in the outpatient clinic and have the current scheduling staff arrange the appointments. On *who* can do the evaluations, it turns out the insurance regulations do not reimburse if the anesthesia staff do the evaluations, but they pay if it is performed by other clinical staff."

COO: "You know, we have some excess capacity in the hospitalist program in the utilization of its nurse practitioners and physician assistants. Any reason we couldn't use them with the right education and protocols?"

Anesthesia chair: "That's perfect. I can have the protocols and an educational orientation program ready for them within two weeks. How soon can we get access to the clinic rooms?"

COO: "If you can do two weeks, so can I. Let's aim to put this plan into action in two weeks and develop a communication plan by tomorrow so the team will know what we are doing and why."

Anesthesia chair: "Done!"

NEGOTIATION STEPS

The above dialogue is an excellent example of using objective data to not only define the problem but also craft a solution to it. It also shows how the concept of inventing options for mutual gain can be put to work. To further illustrate, let's move on to the actual steps for negotiating the resolution of expectations. As mentioned earlier, there are three discrete but related steps in the negotiation process:

1. Discover your expectations.
2. Discover their expectations.
3. Invent options for mutual gain.

You and your staff need to know each of these steps and be skilled at using them as appropriate, depending on the needs of the situation. Let's look at each step.

Negotiation Step 1: Discovering Expectations—Yours

In a customer service text, it may seem curious to start negotiations by discovering your expectations instead of starting with the patient. However, it is important for you and your staff to recognize that everyone approaches each healthcare encounter with expectations of their own. As we note in Chapter 2, the first source of expectation is from answering the question, "Is this a patient, or is this a customer?" But staff have other sets of expectations as well. What are their expectations for this specific clinical encounter? What percent patient or percent customer are they serving? They need to ask themselves, *Is this really the right patient for me, for this unit, for this segment of healthcare?* Just as you consider which negotiation strategy you will use when you enter a meeting, your staff must think of negotiation strategies regarding their expectations for the clinical encounters they have.

In discovering our expectations, several concepts are helpful for healthcare workers to consider, including the following:

- What is my stress tolerance level (STL)?
- How stressful has the shift been so far?
- What are my hot buttons?
- How many hours/patients are left in the shift?
- What are my *specific* expectations for *this* patient?
- Am I ready to be open-minded, unstressed, and "at the top of my game" with this patient?

Understand Distress, Eustress, and the Stress Tolerance Level

In addition to assessing expectations for the next meeting, the next negotiation, or the next patient, staff would be wise to assess where they are on their own stress tolerance curve (a concept we learned from a friend and colleague, Joan Kyes, RN). We tend to think of stress as bad, but not all stress is truly negative, as Hans Selye (1978) demonstrated in his research nearly 30 years ago. It takes a certain amount of stress—positive stress, called *eustress* in Selye's model—to motivate us, to get us out of bed in the morning, to move us forward in our careers, to get us to pursue further education, to get us to go to the *n*th meeting of the day, to meet with the disgruntled medical staff member or employee.

It is only when stress reaches, in Malcom Gladwell's phrase, "the tipping point"—when it goes over the top and becomes *distress*—that it assumes the characteristic of negative stress, the more common meaning of the term *stress* (Gladwell 2002). That's the point at which we reach our STL. The question then becomes, "Are you capable of the self-knowledge and self-reflection required to understand what you look like, what you feel like, as you approach the limits of your STL?" For example, what warning signals do you experience when you think to yourself, *If one more person with one more problem or one more complaint comes whining to me, I'm going to . . .* scream, yell, cry, jump out the window, choke them—whatever your response is to distress or negative stress?

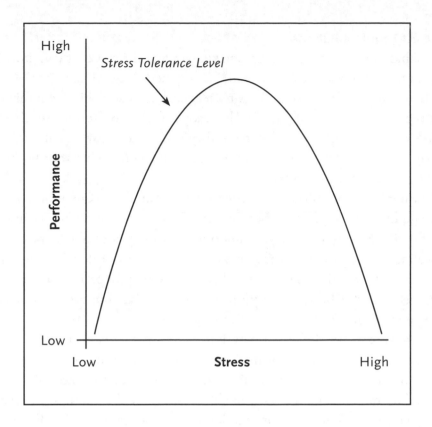

Train yourself to know when you're reaching your STL. Does your pulse go up, your face blush, your stomach churn, your palms sweat? Whatever it is that you look like and feel like—and it is different for each individual—figure it out ahead of time so you'll know your profile as you approach your STL (and before anyone else reaches theirs). One of the best ways to discover what you are like as you approach your STL is to use your colleagues as a barometer. If you have the courage to ask them and they have the courage (and your permission) to answer honestly, trust us, they know what you look and act like as you approach your STL.

Now, what should you do when you are approaching your STL? Decompress, de-stress, take a time out, close the door, turn off the lights, lie on the floor, put on some music, think pleasant thoughts, meditate, look at a picture of your family— whatever is needed to step back from the precipice of your STL. Again, it varies for each individual, but you should know what it takes to rebuild your reservoir of stress acceptance, to come back down to the left side of the curve shown in the graph above. Don't take on the next challenge facing you—whether it is a tough negotiation as a healthcare leader or a tough set of expectations from a patient or family—without de-stressing, to the best extent possible, prior to entering the negotiation.

Disconnect Your Hot Buttons

Everyone has hot buttons. Not everyone knows what theirs are. If you don't know what your hot buttons are, ask your staff, just as you did regarding your STL—they know. If you are familiar with 360-degree feedback, think of this as a mini version of that type of assessment. If you're really ready for a hot-button reality check, ask your spouse, significant other, children—they *really* know how to push your buttons—or other family members. It's important to recognize what your hot buttons are prior to negotiating expectations.

Following the mini-360-degree feedback process and subsequent introspection, you should know what your hot buttons are. Now disconnect them. Mentally put yourself in an encounter where your hot buttons would normally be pushed: perhaps dealing with a particularly troublesome direct report or department manager or speaking with the shrill family member of an unhappy patient. Imagine your response as your hot buttons are pushed—the negative, nonproductive ways in which you fail to invent options for mutual gain.

Now "rewind"; take the scenario back to the start. Mentally envision the stress of the hot-button situation—but this time, envision yourself not reacting in your normal hot-button way. See yourself handling the situation gracefully, hear the charm and dignity in your voice as you defuse this difficult situation, and feel how relaxed you are as the negotiation unfolds with equanimity. You've disconnected your hot button. You've learned how to handle the situation differently. Now do it for all the rest of your hot buttons.

Avoid Counting Down—Using Creative Energy to Power Through

In thinking about the number of hours or patients or meetings or problems left in the shift or business day, you are consciously or subconsciously assessing your energy reserves. Most healthcare professionals are familiar with the concept of "counting down," whereby many B-Team members pace themselves (so they rationalize) over the course of their day. It is particularly prominent at the end of the day, when the willingness to take on new work—new patients—goes dramatically south. Their mental model for this is, "Well, I am going off duty in an hour, so it really wouldn't be fair for me to pick up new patients just to pass them off to someone else." Of course, the problem with this rationalization is that the patients' needs become secondary to the staff's needs. (Remember Rule 1 [always do the right thing for the patient] and Rule 2 [do the right thing for those who take care of the patient] from the BestPractices mission statement.)

Before you know it, instead of counting down one hour prior to the end of the shift, it's two hours, then three. In more than 30 years as emergency physicians, we have seen some of our B-Team comrades start counting down *before they even get to the ED to 'work' their shift!*

Joan Kyes had a wonderful concept that she called "creative energy," which allows us to creatively invest our energy by completing tasks in a timely fashion and puts the energy at our disposal for future projects. Joan stated that we all have had the experience of being around people who seem to have an inexhaustible reservoir of energy—they are always willing to take on the next challenge. Others always seem to have "nothing left in the tank" when it comes to their energy reservoir.

Joan made the point, bolstered by Hans Selye (1978) and Erik Erickson (1980) (but we believe the formulation was uniquely hers), that all of us have basically the same energy reservoir with roughly the same amount of energy in it. When we take on a new project of any sort, we take an "energy packet," as Joan called it, from the reservoir for the effort at hand. The size of the energy packet varies depending on the magnitude of the project. (To be sure, it also depends on experience with the problem at hand. As historian David McCullough said about President Harry S Truman, "Courage is having done it before.")

The energy doesn't return to the energy reservoir until the project has been completed and the packet is closed and returned to the reservoir. Thus, people who appear to have low energy levels are usually those who have multiple energy packets out and open, depleting their reservoir. Those folks don't need a can of 5-Hour Energy; they need to close their energy packets and get them back in the reservoir. It takes creativity to close those packets in a timely fashion in order to put that energy at our disposal for future projects.

In undertaking the first step of negotiating by discovering *our* expectations, we should always take a peek at our energy reservoir and close any open packets that we can.

A corollary to the concept of creative energy in terms of B-Team behavior is burnout, a concept that B-Team members turn to as an excuse to practice counting down. They say, "Oh, I'm burned out—I am *so* burned out!" We actually heard one person say, in all seriousness, "I'm suffering from a bad case of *compassion fatigue*"! Compassion fatigue? Joan used to say, "To burn out, you have to catch on fire, and I know a *lot* of people who will never be in danger of burnout by that criterion." (We happen to think that the biggest problem is not "burnout" but rather "rustout." By *rustout* we mean that people have failed to use healthy and effective mechanisms to deal with the stress of the job and instead have defaulted to ineffective and unhealthy coping mechanisms. The "rust" comes from failing to use the effective strategies.)

Identify Your Specific Expectations for *This* Patient or Problem

All of the above steps are helpful in giving us a sense of our basic, overall expectations and how ready we are to put our "game face" on and get to the work of the next patient (or problem, in the case of managers and leaders). But we also need to drill down to the details of the next patient or problem. From a clinical standpoint, as emergency physicians practicing in a busy, high-acuity ED, we have different expectations for each of the following clinical scenarios:

- A major trauma patient being flown in by helicopter
- A patient with fibromyalgia who has been to the ED five times in the last two weeks
- The child with a fever mentioned in Chapter 3
- An ICU (intensive care unit) patient straight out of the OR with multiple lines and drips
- The ICU "patient" who should have been transferred to the med/surg floor days ago who presses his call button about 14 times per hour

As we discuss earlier in the book, our staff at least tacitly go through the "Are they patients, or are they customers?" diagnosis, but they also have a mental model of what their expectations are for that next patient before they ever walk into the room. Those expectations vary from person to person by background, training, and experience. They are not right or wrong—but they are very much *there* and form an important part of our ability to negotiate the resolution of expectations. What is "wrong" is not recognizing our expectations and taking them into account in each and every patient interaction. We need to train our staff to do this, as very few of them have been taught this process.

For leaders and managers, there is wisdom to developing expectations when we approach our team members in trying to solve problems or address opportunities. Before going into a meeting or speaking with key members of our team, we should always take a few moments to think about our expectations, as well as what success might look like as we negotiate to resolve expectations among the team. The principles of intrinsic motivation and keeping the end in mind (discussed in Chapter 1) are also core principles to adhere to when discovering our own expectations.

Negotiation Step 2: Discovering Expectations—Theirs

How can you discover the expectations of those with whom you negotiate—whether they are your colleagues, the medical staff, or patients? Two simple words suffice:

Ask them.

The vast majority of the time, a straightforward, nonconfrontational question—*What are your expectations?*—gets a straightforward, nonconfrontational answer. While we sometimes need to help others discover their expectations through a series of nearly Socratic questions (What would success look like to you in this project? How can we best take into account our employees' expectations? How would you like me to handle your concerns?), we can usually clarify expectations without much inquiry. Nonetheless, *how* we ask can be a source of interest, particularly in clinical encounters.

Emergency physician to patient: "What's wrong with you?"

Patient to emergency physician: "You're the doctor, you're supposed to know. That's why I came here."

Healthcare provider to patient: "What brings you here today?"

Patient to healthcare provider: "The bus."

I once picked up an ED chart and astutely read the nurses' note—why not take advantage of our nursing colleagues' insights on the patient prior to going in the room?—which read, "Patient states he fell out of a tree."

Walking in the room, I extended my hand and, with a warm smile, said, "Mr. Smith, I'm Dr. Mayer. I'm the emergency physician who will be caring for you today. I understand from the nurses' note that you fell out of a tree. What did you hit when you landed?"

He replied, "The ground, Newton!"

That incident happened more than 15 years ago, but it taught me to be a little clearer in my questions regarding expectations. (Incidentally, after considerable reflection on this matter, I don't think it was "the ground" that bothered me—I think it was "Newton!" Clearly, this was an educated man who understood the laws of physics. After all, he didn't say "Einstein" or "Dumbo.") Notwithstanding that little bon mot, I have found it best to negotiate from a clear understanding of the patient's expectation by asking simple questions such as, "What are your expectations?" or "How can I help you?"

Establishing Expectations, Creating Patient Loyalty

As important as it is to establish clearly what the patients' expectations are, as we have already seen, our ultimate goal is not just to *meet* expectations but to *exceed* them whenever possible. It is when we consistently exceed expectations that we are able to create and sustain patients' loyalty. As we are discovering the patient's expectations, we can begin to establish loyalty through the language we use. Here are examples:

- "What's the most important thing I can do to not only meet but exceed your expectations?"
- "What's the most important thing I can do to make this a highly successful emergency visit?"
- "What's the most important thing we can do today to help you recover from your surgery?"

Obviously, at every stage of the experience, wherever the patient is in touching the healthcare system, you can substitute the appropriate phrase in the examples above. The key is that while there are always similarities among patients with the same problem, each patient is different and each patient will verbalize her expectations in her own unique way.

In addition to asking how we can create loyal patients by exceeding expectations, we can use whiteboards in the patients' rooms so that not only do the patient and family know who the caregivers are but the "most important thing" is captured and visibly noted, as shown here.

> Individual Patient Care
>
> Doctor—Jennifer Jones, MD
> Nurse—Brian
> Tech—Sally
> What's the most important thing we can do for you today?—Help me start walking after my surgery.

Restate Expectations

To obtain the maximum clarity regarding expectations, it is wise to restate the expectations in simple, clear language after you have heard them.

> *CEO to department director:* "What I heard you say is that your department is different and therefore shouldn't be held to the same service excellence standards as the rest of the team. Did I hear you correctly?"

Lab director to vice president of medical affairs: "OK, it is my understanding that 'success' in this matter means that 95 percent of STAT laboratory requests will be completed in 20 minutes or less. Is that correct?"

Chief nurse executive to nursing managers: "I heard you say that nurse recruitment and retention would improve dramatically if we could deliver on a commitment to no more than four patients at any one time for any medical/surgical nurse. Is that correct?"

If we are discovering the expectations of our team members in addressing problems or exploiting opportunities, keep in mind that those expectations are often a "moving target" and should never be assumed, even if we have dealt with those precise team members before. Heed the wisdom that four-time NCAA National Championship Coach Mike Krzyzewski shared with me in 2013:

> Things don't stay the same. You have to understand that not only your situation changes, but the people you are working with aren't the same day-to-day. Someone is sick. Someone is having a wedding. You must gauge the mood, the thinking level of the team that day.

What is Coach K's offensive philosophy? What does he call his signature way of having his teams play defense? What's his view on the zone press? It's a bit of a trick question, because as Coach K has been the first to say, he doesn't have a concrete, set-in-stone philosophy in *any* of these areas. But he is deeply committed to discovering each year what the strengths and weaknesses of his team are, and he builds around them. The same should be true of healthcare leaders.

Your job is to discover the team's expectation each day in each situation. Never assume. Always explore. One of the keys is for the leader to connect the team to its purpose as a core part of discovering its expectations of the problem or opportunity.

Connecting our healthcare professionals and staff with their core purpose is an essential step in helping them discover their expectations, and it is a concept that many great minds have championed, including Warren Bennis, Peter Drucker, Quint Studer, and Tom Peters. Connecting "the prose and the passion" and helping your staff discover where their deep joy meets the world's deep needs keep the focus on collective and individual expectations regarding the success of the effort.

> Only connect!
> That was the whole of her sermon.
> Only connect the prose and the passion, and both will be exalted.
> And human love will be seen at its highest.
> Live in fragments no longer.
> Only connect . . .
> —E. M. Forster, *Howards End*

Negotiation Step 3: Invent Options for Mutual Gain

Once you have a clear sense of your expectations in the service encounter and discovered the patient's, family's, or staff's expectations, you need to assess ways in which these expectations differ, since this is the point from which negotiations will proceed. For example, in the "Are they patients, or are they customers" exercise, we found that the lady with a heart attack was, in the healthcare workers' estimation, a patient. Here, then, is the question: *Does she agree with you?*

The answer is "Yes" because the sicker she is, the more horizontal she is, and the more likely she (and her family) is to agree with your customer service diagnosis. This is an example of where expectations are likely similar or congruous, and less negotiation is needed.

But what about the three-year-old child at 3:00 a.m. with the fever? Do the parents agree that their child is more of a customer, or more vertical? Absolutely not. Clearly they think the child is a patient, nearly horizontal. Now it becomes a situation that involves negotiation.

Obviously, telling the parents they have unreasonable expectations isn't going to work. Nor is saying any of the following (all of which are drawn from real conservations with patients):

"You're not the sickest patient here."

"This isn't really a fever."

"What are you wasting my time for?"

"You came to the ED for *this*?"

These statements not only don't work but they make the situation much worse. So does the following comment, made in response to a patient who said to his nurse, "But I'm in pain!" Her reply? "Honey, we're *all* in pain here."

Instead, *invent options for mutual gain*. Exhibit 5.1 offers examples of how combining communication skills and inventing options for mutual gain can work to the mutual benefit of all.

If we are going to ask our staff to negotiate all day, every day—and we are, make no mistake about it—we need to invest in them and their success by teaching them the skills, abilities, tools, and techniques of negotiation. Make it a part of both orientation and ongoing education. After all, when you make a list of your best A-Team members, don't be surprised if they are also your best negotiators.

Exhibit 5.1: Examples of Inventing Options for Mutual Gain

Patient/Family/Staff Issue	Option Offered
"But I'm in pain—can't you give me something to take it away?"	"We expect you to have some pain in the postoperative period, particularly on the first day. But your patient-controlled anesthesia pump is designed to give you control of your pain without giving you too much medication."
"What did my CT scan show?"	"Your doctor is seeing patients in the office. Let me see if she or her nurse (or nurse practitioner or physician's aide) can talk to the radiologist and let you know before she comes by on rounds this evening."
"I have to wait for the specialist?"	"We think your case requires the input of a specialist in this area. But I'll check to see when she's coming and make sure all the data are ready and available. Is there anything else I can do to help?"
"I can't go home from the hospital until 6 p.m. I don't have a ride and my family is at work."	"I've arranged for you to be cared for in our Discharge Lounge while you wait for your family. You'll be more comfortable there."
"It's unreasonable to hold our unit to service standards when we're so short staffed."	[As the CEO] "Both staffing and service excellence are core competencies I expect from our leaders. We can track satisfaction scores by provider to assess agency versus permanent staff. Most important is to remember that the number one reason for service excellence is that it makes all our jobs easier, not harder!"

SURVIVAL SKILLS SUMMARY

- In healthcare, we negotiate all day, every day—with patients, families, and our team members—and yet most of us have never had a formal course in negotiating.
- Negotiation is an interactive process between two or more people designed to achieve a desired outcome through effective communication.
- Keep in mind that
  - The best **negotiators** are the best **learners.**
  - The best **learners** are the best **listeners.**
  - Therefore, the best **negotiators** are the best **listeners.**

- In communications among people, only 7 percent is verbal content—the rest is vocal expression and visual cues.
- Active listening is an extremely effective communication tool in which the listener systematically feeds back what the speaker has heard the listener say in order to
  - improve clarity of the message,
  - make listening a participative process, and
  - ensure common ground is gained in the ongoing process of communication.
- Define success before the negotiation begins.
- In *Getting to Yes,* Fisher, Ury, and Patton (1991) stress four key negotiating principles:
  1. Separate the people from the problem.
  2. Focus on interests and principles, not positions.
  3. Invent options for mutual gain.
  4. Insist on prospective, objective criteria by which to define success.
- Always make it "patient first" in any negotiation.
- Follow these Survival Skill expectation negotiation steps:
  1. Discover your expectations.
  2. Discover the patient's expectations.
  3. Invent options for mutual gain.
- Investing in negotiation training for healthcare staff is one of the wisest commitments a leader can make.

REFERENCES

Berry, L. L., and K. D. Seltman. 2008. *Leadership Lessons from Mayo Clinic: Inside One of the World's Most Respected Service Organizations.* New York: McGraw-Hill.

Covey, S. 2013. *The 7 Habits of Highly Effective People: Powerful Lessons in Personal Change*, 25th anniversary ed. New York: Simon & Schuster.

Erikson, E. 1980. *Identity and the Life Cycle.* New York: Norton.

Fisher, R., W. Ury, and B. Patton. 1991. *Getting to Yes: Negotiating Agreement Without Giving In*, 2nd ed. New York: Penguin.

Gladwell, M. 2002. *The Tipping Point: How Little Things Can Make a Big Difference.* San Francisco: Back Bay Books.

Groopman, J. 2007. *How Doctors Think.* Boston: Houghton Mifflin.

Mayer, T. A., J. Kaplan, R. W. Strauss, and R. J. Cates. 2014. "Customer Service in Emergency Medicine." In *Strauss and Mayer's Emergency Department Management,* edited by R. Strauss and T. Mayer. New York: McGraw-Hill.

Mehrabian, A. 1981. *Silent Messages: Implicit Communication of Emotions and Attitude.* Chicago: Aldine-Atherton.

Selye, H. 1978. *The Stress of Life.* New York: McGraw-Hill.

MORE RESOURCES ON NEGOTIATION IN SERVICE EXCELLENCE

Marcus, L. J., B. C. Dorn, and E. J. McNulty. 2011. *Renegotiating Healthcare: Resolving Conflict to Build Collaboration,* 2nd ed. San Francisco: Jossey-Bass.

Ury, W. 1999. *Getting to Peace: Transforming Conflict at Home, at Work, and in the World.* New York: Penguin.

———. 1993. *Getting Past No: Negotiating Your Way from Confrontation to Cooperation.* New York: Bantam.

The best of the books on negotiation, all of which are very practical.

Frieberg, K., and J. Frieberg. 1997. *Nuts! Southwest Airlines' Crazy Recipe for Business and Personal Success.* New York: Broadway Books.

Gitomer, J. 1998. *Customer Satisfaction Is Worthless, Customer Loyalty Is Priceless: How to Make Customers Love You, Keep Them Coming.* Austin, TX: Bard Press.

Each of these books is excellent and contains good sections on service recovery.

Mayer, T., and R. J. Cates. 1999. "Service Excellence in Health Care." *Journal of the American Medical Association* 282 (13): 1281–83.

Mayer, T. A., R. J. Cates, M. J. Mastorovich, and D. L. Royalty. 1998. "Emergency Department Patient Satisfaction: Customer Service Training Improves Patient Satisfaction and Ratings of Physician and Nurse Skill." *Journal of Healthcare Management* 43 (5): 427–40.

These articles are two of the contributions we've made to the literature.

CHAPTER 6

Survival Skill 3: Creating Moments of Truth

The idea of "moments of truth" is not our invention; indeed, many have claimed the concept as their own. We've all heard the adage, "Great ideas have many parents." But the original description of this important concept came from Jan Carlzon's 1987 book, *Moments of Truth*. Carlzon was a former CEO of Scandinavian Airways, who had assumed that position at the age of 39, at a time when the airline was in serious trouble on all fronts. In resuscitating the airline's reputation for service excellence, Carlzon (1987) addressed the employees in the following (paraphrased) way:

> You, the employees of Scandinavian Airways, have been defining the airline as a certain number and type of plane, with specified revenue capacity, specified load capacity, taking off and landing on time, with the passengers' bags getting to the right place.
>
> I don't believe that's the way the airline is defined. I believe that the airline is defined by 50,000 Moments of Truth a day. A Moment of Truth occurs when you—the employees of Scandinavian Airways—have contact with those we serve—the people who fly the airline and their friends and family. Thus, each of you defines the airline on a daily basis by these 50,000 Moments of Truth.

In Carlzon's definition, a moment of truth occurs whenever service employees have an encounter with those they serve. So what? What's the implication for healthcare?

Gather your staff. After defining *moments of truth* for them along Carlzon's lines, address your staff with this question: "Do you think our patients have any idea how many beds we have in this institution? How many nurses we have? How many doctors? How many cardiovascular surgeons? No. Of course not, but they know you."

Carlzon's message is as simple as this: *From the customers' perspective, the people performing the service are the company.*

In *The Little Big Things: 163 Ways to Pursue Excellence,* Tom Peters (2010) takes the moments-of-truth concept to a new level when he states, "[O]ur goal, perhaps our primary goal, in every flavor and every size of business, is to MTMMOT—Manage to Memorable Moments of Truth."

We should *hire for* people who can create moments of truth, *promote and reward* people who have created moments of truth, and *make leaders of* those who exemplify this trait through their actions.

In the movie *All That Jazz!* renowned choreographer and dancer Bob Fosse is played by Roy Scheider. Throughout the movie, just before going onstage to dance, Scheider's character looks in the dressing room mirror and says, "It's showtime, folks!" Well, in healthcare it is always showtime, and it is high time we made sure all of our folks know it. Healthcare, particularly for physicians and nurses, is *performance art,* and we need to be performance artists. (We say more about how to hire for the performance artist trait in Chapter 13.) And, as we discuss earlier, in healthcare all of us are onstage all the time.

VISION, MISSION, AND VALUES

The patients/customers in your healthcare system can't know you or even your leadership and management team to any meaningful degree. But they do know those on the front lines—and they will judge *your* service by *their* service. If those on the front line create positive moments of truth (through A-Team behaviors), your institution will have a great reputation for service throughout the community.

Moments of truth lead to exceeding expectations and are directly tied to patient loyalty. This chain starts with your staff understanding the importance of A-Team behaviors and the destructive nature of B-Team behaviors. It continues when they understand and embrace their role as service providers.

In other words, they must be servant leaders, as described by Robert Greenleaf (2002). They must have a servant's heart; they must know that a part of their deep joy is in meeting the deep needs of others, particularly at the patients' and families' most desperate times. Here's the simplest exposition of Greenleaf's (2002) concept of servant leadership:

Do those served grow as persons? Do they, while being served, become healthier, wiser, freer, more autonomous, more likely themselves to become servants? And, what is the effect on the least privileged in society?

A simple litmus test by which to gauge staff's inclination toward servant leadership is to ask the following questions:

1. Do these staff members grow as people in the course of delivering care?
2. Are they more likely to become servants themselves?

But it is up to you to convey to your staff just how important service is to you, as a leader of the institution. That importance undoubtedly is reflected in your institution's mission and vision statements. But do your actions back up those words, consistently and visibly?

Let's revisit the idea of these organizational statements for purposes of this discussion: It is our view that mission, vision, and values statements must be direct, simple, and easily remembered. Too often these statements drone on and lack "punch." If you can't say it in 30 seconds and the person you're saying it to can't repeat it back in 15 seconds, it's too long and complicated. Seth Godin, an author and a leadership mentor, agrees, as he shared with us in 2012:

If you can't describe your position in 8 words or less, you don't have a position.

What's the mission statement for our physician group, BestPractices?

BestPractices Exists to Create an Innovative Future through:

- The **SCIENCE** of Clinical Excellence
- The **ART** of Customer Service
- The **BUSINESS** of Execution

Simple. Clear. Easily remembered. Easy to deliver on? Hardly. But at least every one of our team members has a clear sense of why we are there. Who designed this mission statement? Our entire physician team participated, since it had to be *their* mission statement, not ours. Remember the old saying, "If they are not with you on the takeoff, they won't be with you on the landing"? Give staff a hand in designing their own mission statement, and they are far more likely to embrace it.

Everything we do is measured against how well it serves the needs expressed by the mission. In our company, if an activity doesn't serve these needs, it doesn't add value. The third part of the credo, the business of execution, is critical. The idea is that anyone can have a good idea, but only world-class organizations and great leaders can execute that idea—or any idea. As Ben Franklin is said to have commented, "Well done is better than well said."

So the BestPractices mission statement is a little over Godin's eight-word limit, but it is a fundamentally terse statement that carries a lot of meaning. It is powerful enough that the billion-dollar company with which we merged, EmCare, adopted it as its own statement.

Furthermore, it is not the mission statement on the wall but the service provided in the institution that is important. As we indicate in the previous chapter, *better to have one person practicing empowered customer service than a hundred posted mission statements proclaiming it.*

In our emergency department (ED), we have had the pleasure of working with many customer service champions, among them doctors, nurses, administrators, and essential services staff. But three people stand out: Felicia, Fannie, and Bernardo.

Felicia and Fannie are runners who take radiology films from the ED to the radiologists to be read, after which they return the films to the ED. Bernardo works in housekeeping. By the measuring stick of years of formal education, they may have the least in our department. But from the benchmark of customer service, they are at the top of the heap. They are unfailingly pleasant, kind, thoughtful, and generous—not just to the patients but to their teammates as well. They have the quintessential servant's heart. When they are on duty, everyone is a little happier, regardless of how high the volume, acuity, or stress levels may be. They exemplify the A-Team.

What's the point? You've got people just like them in your hospital. Make sure you and your managers know who they are. Turn your Bernardos, Felicias, and Fannies loose, and others will follow them. Reward your service champions, and celebrate their success.

It is important to remember that service excellence is elusive: It is impermanent and evanescent. It cannot outlast the customer encounter unless a meaningful moment of truth has been created. Like fitness or conditioning, you can't achieve it and then declare victory, to be fit evermore. Service excellence has to occur every day, every night, in every unit throughout your institution—your goal must be excellent service provided 24/7/365. That's hard, because the battle is never over; it's always anew. *In service excellence, there is no finish line—the victory is in the running.*

MOMENTS OF TRUTH—THE NORDSTROM STORY

Without question, Nordstrom is one of the world's leaders in the retail industry. Its reputation is widely known and, in the estimation of many, justly deserved. Its service successes are detailed in at least two books: *The Nordstrom Way,* by Robert Spector and Patrick McCarthy (1995), and *Fabled Service,* by Betsy Sanders (1995). Sanders rose up through the ranks of the Nordstrom organization, eventually becoming a motivational speaker on the principles she learned at that company, as detailed in her book. The book is so good that we actually bought it by the case for our ED staff when we began our service excellence journey.

But the problem with service is that it isn't permanent and it is always unique to the individual encounter. To illustrate, here's a story that we tell at our seminars. We invite you to share it with others. Other than the name of the salesman, it is an actual experience I (RJC) had at a Nordstrom store.

When we first began teaching these courses, my oldest daughter, Beth, decided that I needed to look a bit spiffier if I was going to be speaking to sophisticates such as yourselves. At the time, Beth worked for an insurance company, the executives of which were as sharply dressed as you could imagine.

So Beth said, "Dad, you need to go and get a really nice suit where our executives shop—Nordstrom." At the time, I was getting my clothes from a very nice store called Britches (since closed), but the store leaned a little more toward sport coats and casual slacks than finely tailored suits. In fact, the Britches pants I was wearing at the time were not to Beth's liking—she said they were too big and too baggy and they looked like clown pants. Those pants might have looked good on a younger man, a taller man, a thinner man, a more athletic man (some kind of man that Dad was not), but to Beth they looked like clown pants. So she said, "Go to Nordstrom, get a new suit, and you'll look great!"

I went to Nordstrom, dressed fairly casually, where a salesman, Mr. Smith (not his real name), greeted me and began to assist. I told him three things I ordinarily don't say to people upon first meeting them. First, I told him I was a doctor. I thought he might think I had some discretionary income and might actually be able to afford a Nordstrom suit. Second, I told him that I taught customer service courses—I thought that would really help me get the best of the Nordstrom service experience. Third, I told him I had never been to Nordstrom before, so here was a chance for him to capture a customer for life with the legendary Nordstrom service. I thought that was the trifecta—I couldn't lose with those three things going for me.

I thought wrong.

Mr. Smith pulled out a beautiful gray suit and said, "Try this nice gray one on— this is a style the executives in this area are very pleased with." I put the suit on and, indeed, it did look nice, but when Mr. Smith looked the other way, I turned the cuff of the jacket over, trying to sneak a peek at the price tag. I saw more zeros than I had ever seen on a piece of clothing in my life. Mr. Smith caught me peeking at the price tag and quickly said, "Oh, that suit looks very nice. It's a Hickey-Freeman; it never goes on sale."

Well, the suit did look nice, and suddenly I heard myself saying something I couldn't believe: "I'll take it!" (I think maybe I was shamed into buying it.) Immediately a tailor came out and began to mark me up to make sure the suit fit perfectly. In the course of measuring the jacket he said, "Did you know that you have one arm longer than the other?" I am over 50 years old and I must admit I did not know that one arm was longer than the other. I couldn't wait until this guy measured my inseam!

The tailor said, "Don't worry, we'll put a shoulder pad on one side and this coat will look spiffy." I'd gone from looking like a clown at Britches to looking spiffy at Nordstrom—well worth the zeros.

Nearly a week later I came back to pick up my spiffy Hickey-Freeman suit, and as luck would have it, Mr. Smith was there, as was the same tailor. It was the night before we were to give one of our customer service talks, and I was excited about getting this new suit. Mr. Smith said, "Just take a few minutes to try it on to make sure it fits." I said, "I'm sure it's fine, there's no need to try it on." But Mr. Smith was insistent—such is the customer service at Nordstrom. I went back into the changing room and put the pants on. Unbelievably, these pants were cut so short that you could see at least four inches of my bare legs above my socks. I shook my head, thinking, "This can't be happening. These must be someone else's pants!" I walked out of the changing room wearing the pants and Mr. Smith looked at me and said, "Put on the coat." I looked at him with fire in my eyes said, "There's no *need* to put on the coat. Look at these pants!"

"Don't worry," he said, "We'll fix the pants. Just put on the coat to see how it fits."

I gave the pants to the tailor, put on my own, and walked out of the dressing room wearing the coat. Looking in the mirror, I realized that the collar was puckered along the entire length of my neck. I turned to the tailor and said, "What is wrong with the collar?"

He said, "It needs pressing."

"If it needed pressing, why didn't you *press* it?" I said.

I then proceeded to cool my heels by gentlemen's ties, while they hurriedly "whittled" on my pants and pressed my coat. The tailor returned in a few minutes and flipped the coat to me like I was some sort of growth on his backside and said, "See if this isn't better." Putting on the coat, I looked at myself in the three-way mirror with the nice bright Nordstrom lights above me and realized that indeed, the collar was now smooth. However, both lapels were now so rippled that they looked like waterfalls on the front of my coat. Another salesman happened to pass by as Mr. Smith was busy with another customer, and I asked him, "What do you think is wrong with this jacket?"

He took one quick glance and said, "Oh, that is flawed. That should have never gotten by the Hickey-Freeman inspectors." Well, I know where the flaw was, and it wasn't at Hickey-Freeman. It was with Moe and Curly in the back. I quickly changed into my clothes, found Mr. Smith, and said, "I am out of here. Keep the suit and give me a refund." He did so, somewhat reluctantly, and as I was walking out of the door, he said, "Please come back—and next time I'll make sure you see our *good* tailor."

Do you think that helped? Of course not; it made the experience worse. Effectively saying "We can't get good help" *never* makes it better.

Nordstrom may be one of the customer service retail leaders—and it is. Betsy Sanders may be evangelical and eloquent about customer service—and she is. Her book may be so good that we bought it by the case and gave it away—and we did. But for me, Nordstrom will forever be that tailor, that salesman, and that suit. It is 100 percent of my experience with Nordstrom. My moment of truth represented service failure, not service excellence. As we said at the outset, *from the customers' perspective, the people performing the service* are *the company.*

Translating Retail Service Excellence to Healthcare Service Excellence

Nordstrom is a service excellence leader in American retailing precisely because this story is the exception, not the rule. No one knows this better than Nordstrom itself. All of this discussion leads us to the critical importance of the people providing the service in healthcare and the concept that *service excellence must be earned with every encounter, every day, 24/7/365.*

Following are some guidelines for instituting a moment-of-truth culture:

◆ Fly the service excellence flag. Make service rounds on the patient care units, and make this activity a protected part of each week—or, even better, each *day*; put it on your schedule and consider it inviolate, such that nothing should make you cancel it.
◆ Insist that your department directors and unit managers follow the same policy. Leaders lead in service by being service champions.
◆ Ask yourself the next time you are in a meeting, "Is this more important than service rounds?"

- Calculate the hourly rate of your team members. Then document how much time they spend in the meeting. At the end of the meeting, multiply the hourly rate of all the participants by the length of the meeting. Then say, "This meeting just cost us $10,000—was it worth it? Or should we have spent it rounding with our teams and our patients?"

♦ Have nursing directors greet each new patient personally, using scripts (discussed later) that help the directors demonstrate a caring attitude. For example, "Please let me know if I can help you" creates a positive expectation, whereas "Please let me know if you have any problems" creates a negative expectation.

♦ Use business cards liberally. Each nurse, physician, physician assistant, and nurse practitioner at BestPractices hospitals has a card with his or her title and name (the nurses' cards show the first name and last initial only, for privacy purposes). They hand these to patients and families, saying, "It's been my pleasure to serve you—please contact me if I can be of help."

♦ Ask patients and families, "What can we do to improve our service?"
  1. "How could we do this better?"
  2. "What needs do you have that we haven't met?"

♦ Tell patients, "I know you have choices in healthcare. We're delighted you chose our hospital."
  - When there are boarders in the ED awaiting an inpatient bed, have the nursing supervisor visit each one and say, "I'm running this hospital tonight. I will find you a bed." Trust us, the beds will be found much more quickly when the supervisor takes this level of personal responsibility.

These are only a few of the hundreds of ways moments of truth can be enacted in your healthcare system.

THE OPEN-BOOK TEST APPROACH TO PATIENT SATISFACTION SURVEYS

Measuring or reporting on patient satisfaction has become a central focus for healthcare institutions. Indeed, it has become an important industry unto itself. Virtually every healthcare system measures patients' satisfaction with inpatient and outpatient services and reports these results to its board of directors. Satisfaction matters, no question about it. However, much of the failure to improve patient satisfaction rates rests on this issue: *Are your surveys a tool, or are they a club?*

In other words, are the scores used as a tool to help you improve your services, your processes, and your employees' skills? Or are the scores used as a club to bludgeon staff with threats and imprecations? Are your department managers saying, "Get those scores up or . . ."? Or what? "We'll fire you"? With current staffing shortages? "We'll make you work harder, longer, for less money"?

No. Start by nurturing a common understanding that measuring patient satisfaction be used as a tool to help make the job easier, not as a punitive measure.

An equally important insight regarding patient satisfaction surveys is best illustrated by a story of my (TM) son Josh. Now a graduate of Dartmouth College and Duke Law with a beautiful wife and two terrific daughters, Josh came home from school one day during his eighth-grade year with a demeanor that could only mean he'd had a bad day. The following father–son conversation occurred:

Dad: Josh, you look like you had a bad day. What happened?

Josh: I had a test and I flunked it.

Dad: Josh, did you know you were going to have this test?

Josh: Of course I did.

As those of you with children know, there are a couple of additional questions a parent is compelled to ask.

Dad: Josh, this test that you knew you were going to have and that you are certain you failed, what sort of test was it?

Josh: It was an open-book test, Dad.

Dad (somewhat stunned)*:* Did you happen to *open the book*, Josh?

Josh: No, Dad. I didn't even take the book to school.

Somehow I resisted the overriding urge to ask the only logical follow-up question: "Josh, do you understand the meaning of 'open-book test'?"

Guess what? *Your patient satisfaction survey is an open-book test.*

All of us know—or could choose to know—the questions on the test before they are asked. Do your staff know what the questions are on your patient satisfaction survey? If not, they're like Josh—the book is right there, waiting to be opened, but they choose not to open it. Use the open-book test approach to patient satisfaction surveys.

Regardless of whether it is HCAHPS (Hospital Consumer Assessment of Healthcare Providers and Systems), Press Ganey, PRC, NRC Picker, or a home-grown survey, it is critical for the staff to take the open-book test approach to make sure we *make the survey work for us instead of us working for the survey.* I (TM) played collegiate football and currently serve as the medical director of the NFL Players Association, so it is perhaps understandable that we draw on a football analogy: the huddle.

Huddle up—1st down: Have the physicians, nurses, and essential services staff each take the survey questions that pertain to them and their areas, and design scripts (see Chapter 12) and processes (see Chapter 15) to not only meet but exceed expectations.

Huddle up—2nd down: Exchange the questions between the different groups. (After all, if we want to know the best A-Team doctor, should we ask the doctors on the unit, or the nurses? The nurses, of course!) Have the groups discuss the A-Team behaviors they see in others and build them into the system of processes you currently have in place.

Huddle up—3rd down: After building in these scripts and A-Team behaviors, systematically hardwire a plan for optimum flow into all processes, adding value and eliminating waste (see Chapter 15).

A Deeper Dive

We are often asked, What do you do on 4th down if things haven't improved? While it is tempting to say, "Back up and punt," the real answer is to begin anew, with more intensity and effort.

While it does not result in a 1st down, punting is intended to give the kicking team better field position, which in turn often leads to victory. In fact, three-time Super Bowl champion coach Joe Gibbs often said that the special teams unit—the players who are on the field for punts, kickoffs and returns, and field goals—"is the key to victory."

The problem for other coaches, of course, is that very *few* people know what Joe Gibbs knows. In healthcare service delivery, you need to be one of those few. Knowing when to take the gains made and secure those gains toward future progress is the key to gaining yardage downfield, or "moving the chains." Here, the "touchdown" in the effort to improve patients' experience is attaining (and sustaining) our targeted scores. These scores are indirect markers of our ability to make the job easier by tying A-Team behaviors and processes to the open-book test approach to patient satisfaction surveys.

This method is framed by a blend of evidence-based language (EBL) and "survey-based language" (SBL), both of which are addressed in more detail in Chapter 12. In devising EBL and SBL, keep this important point in mind: The physicians and nurses are certainly mission-critical to success in creating positive moments of truth—*but so are the rest of the staff.* Anyone who comes into contact with the patient or family is an ambassador for your hospital and healthcare system.

To demonstrate the nature of language, ask your staff the following question:

What do we call departments like radiology and laboratory services?

Almost universally, you will get this answer: Ancillary services.

The term *ancillary,* though, derives from the Latin word *ankilla*, which means "female slave" (I [TM] owe that bit of knowledge to my Latin scholar son, Josh).

All words have meaning.

At our partner hospitals we have banned the term *ancillary* because all of those departments—lab, radiology, scheduling, registration, dietary, environmental services—are anything but ancillary. In fact, they are essential to our ability to safely and effectively care for our patients. So let's call them what they are—*essential services.*

Examples of your open-book "test questions," including the details of HCAHPS questions, are listed in the appendix to this chapter. As you review them, consider the following points. First, research from the Studer Group (see Exhibit 6.1) indicates a strong correlation between ED satisfaction scores (regardless of which survey company is used) and inpatient HCAHPS scores, reflecting the importance of a well-run ED to any hospital.

Second, the HCAHPS survey is not a Likert scale–based survey, with rankings shown on an ordinal scale (usually a 5-point scale in healthcare surveys). Instead, it is an "always, usually, sometimes, never" scale, which is much harder to score well on without a rigorous approach to preparing for the survey, defining specific ways in which scripts and behaviors relate to the questions, and systematically interpreting the survey results (Robinson, Cook, and Studer 2010). As such, the HCAHPS survey has added a new realm to the customer service calculus, since it is more behavior based and less service experience based. By "behavior based," we mean that the questions deal with speed, cleanliness, and quietness. For example, in addition to service-based questions, such as those inquiring about the level of communication and the extent to which staff treat patients with respect, listen carefully, and so forth, it poses the following (CMS 2013):

◆ During this stay, after you pressed the call button, how often did you get help as soon as you wanted it?

Exhibit 6.1: Relationship Between ED and HCAHPS Overall Percentile Rankings

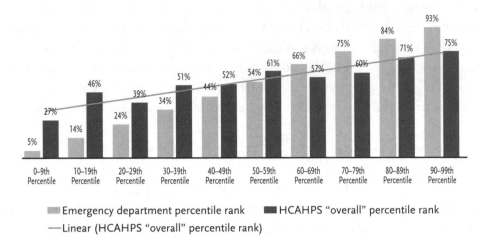

Emergency department percentile rank ▮ HCAHPS "overall" percentile rank
—Linear (HCAHPS "overall" percentile rank)

Source: Reprinted with permission of the Studer Group.

◆ How often did you get help in getting to the bathroom or in using a bedpan as soon as you wanted?
◆ How often were your room and bathroom kept clean?
◆ How often was the area around your room kept quiet at night?

As of 2014, the final version of the Emergency Department Comprehensive Assessment of Healthcare Providers and Services (EDCAHPS) will also be administered, with the expectation that some portion of ED facility reimbursement will be tied to these results.

Final Thoughts on the Open-Book Test Approach to Surveys

Clearly, the importance of taking the open-book test approach is difficult to overstate. Access to the updated list of HCAHPS questions (and, eventually, the EDCAHPS questions) is available at the Hospital Compare website (www.hospitalcompare.hhs. gov). Select "About the Data" and then "Survey of patients' experiences" (CMS 2013).

Survey scoring is, by nature, a moving target in that the discrete data points from the results will move over time as the questions and the scales change. That said, hardwiring a strong customer service culture into your organization will help ensure service excellence and, thereby, high customer satisfaction scores regardless of how the survey scales shift.

Most surveys include questions relating specifically to doctors, nurses, laboratory, radiology, and so on. It's generally a good idea to have each segment of the care delivery team review these particular questions and come up with its own A-Team behaviors and scripts. However, it is also a good idea to circulate those responses among the various areas of care delivery so that, for example, nurses review doctors' questions, doctors review nurses' questions, nurses review the radiology-specific questions, and so forth. This is truly a team approach to the open-book test.

MOMENTS OF TRUTH—TEAMWORK

Throughout healthcare, the importance of teamwork is regularly emphasized. If you ask anyone in the healthcare field if he and his colleagues are a team, that person will likely answer along the lines of, "Oh, yes. Team, team, team. See the poster on the wall that says we are?"

Of course, posters and slogans do not make a team. We believe you can spend an hour on any healthcare unit in the United States and tell by the interactions between the people whether they operate as a team or not. Teamwork is one of the fundamental pieces of success in healthcare customer service. *The number one reason to get customer service right is that it makes the job easier through A-Team behaviors and A-Team attitudes.* The A-Team makes work easier.

Several years ago, we had the honor and privilege of spending a weekend aboard the nuclear aircraft carrier USS *George Washington,* which was a truly transformational experience. Among the many lessons we learned from observing the men and women serving on the carrier, the most informative were the demonstrations of their commitment to teamwork. The 4.5 acres comprising the flight deck of a nuclear aircraft carrier is the most dangerous territory on Earth. Fighter and attack jets, fully armed with ordnance, are catapulted off a deck splashed with oil and seawater, accelerating from a standstill to 150 miles per hour in less than two seconds by catapults powered by 2 million horsepower. Aircraft are recovered in cycles at the opposite end of the flight deck by other members of the team, each with specific duties. The roar is deafening, even with earplugs and protective headgear, so communications among the team are accomplished by an elaborate yet widely understood set of hand signals. Each step of the choreography interrelates closely with the others, from raising the aircraft off the hangar deck via elevators to the flight deck to positioning the aircraft in an elegant series of moves to the catapult and through their explosive launch. The flight deck crew wear brightly colored shirts, each color denoting their role on the team, including red for the ordnance crew (the folks who load the bombs and missiles), white for safety officers, green for catapult and recovery wire operators, yellow for launch personnel (the "shooters"), and silver flame-proof suits for the elite fire and recovery team.

We asked to see the training manuals describing the elaborate ballet of personnel and machinery. Sheepishly, the captain replied, "We don't have one. These procedures are passed down verbally—and accurately—among our crew."

Their extraordinary level of teamwork is a benchmark that all of us in healthcare can aspire to. But short of painstakingly passing down instructions with extraordinary and consistent accuracy, how can we train for teamwork and communicate its importance? Consider the following story, told to us by legendary college football coach Lou Holtz, as you contemplate your answer.

I was scheduled to give a talk not far from Charlotte, North Carolina, one night, but as luck would have it, my plane arrived late on this rainy evening. I dashed off in the rental car and drove further and further into the hills of North Carolina on the rain-soaked roads.

Fortunately, the rain stopped, but I was still running late, and as I looked over to check the map, I slid off the road into a ditch, where my rental car was mired helplessly in the mud. But today was my lucky day! A farmer emerged out of the mist on the road, and he was leading a huge, old plow horse he called Buddy. I waved the farmer down and asked if he could help me. The old fellow looked at me, looked at my car, and looked back at Buddy—and then he said, "Yep, I believe I can help you. You get in the car, put it into neutral, and steer."

He pulled out a rope and tied it to the front bumper of my car, looped it around Buddy's harness, and tied it tightly. Cupping his hands around his mouth, he yelled, "Pull, Nellie, Pull!" Nothing happened.

Then he yelled, "Pull, Rosie, Pull!" Nothing happened.

Then he yelled, "Pull, Buster, Pull!" Nothing happened.

Then, softly, he said, "Pull, Buddy, pull."

That old horse pulled my car out of the ditch in nothing flat. My car was sitting high and dry, and I was ready to get on the road and make it to my speech. As the farmer was untying the rope from under the car and around Buddy's harness, I couldn't help but ask him, "Sir, it's none of my business, but I just noticed that you called your horse by the wrong name three times. What gives?"

The old farmer looked at me and said, "Well, you see, old Buddy is blind. And if he thought he was the only one pulling, he wouldn't even try."

It's good to have a team, but sometimes we just have to get our old, blind Buddy pulling in the right direction.

MOMENTS OF TRUTH—THE STAR THROWER

You and your staff are involved in one of the greatest endeavors one could hope for—delivering healthcare to those in need. It is an honored and honorable calling, and each of us represents a piece of the teamwork of delivering that care. It is essential that your staff understand how deeply you honor what they do.

How do you communicate it? There are many ways, but we have found the following story to be one of the most effective in demonstrating your regard for them. It is, on its surface, a hokey story, appealing to the deepest emotions and brightest lights of your staff. However, its effectiveness makes any discomfort worthwhile. It was inspired by a wonderful and incisive essay titled "The Star Thrower," by scientist Dr. Loren Eiseley (1978). Here's how we tell it.

I should warn you at the outset that the following story is probably apocryphal and certainly sentimental, if not outright hokey. But it's good enough that I'll risk telling it to you anyway.

In our area near Washington, D.C., many people need to take vacations for rest and relaxation. A lot of them go to the Outer Banks, the barrier islands off the North Carolina coast, which are a several-hour drive away. The story is told that a businessman from our nation's capital decided to take his family, rent a house at the Outer Banks, and unwind at the beach. He checked in on a Saturday afternoon and settled his family in. As it turned out, that Saturday night there was a huge storm that howled in off the Atlantic. The storm created a significant tidal surge, such that water came up and underneath the house he was renting. But as you may know, these houses are built on stilts, so the tide simply washed up under the house and then went back out to sea.

But a curious thing happened during that tidal surge. It carried so many starfish with it that, when the businessman walked out of his rented house on Sunday morning, it appeared that every starfish in the sea had been deposited on the beaches of the Outer Banks. Truly, it appeared that the sky had "rained starfish." It was early in the morning, and the man looked to his left and looked to his right prior to walking down the beach. In the distance off to his left he saw someone, so he walked in that direction. As he did so, he became curious, as the figure on the beach repeatedly bent over and then stood back up, bent over and then stood back up, over and over. As he walked further in that direction, he became even more curious, because he realized it was a little girl, about nine years old. She was picking up starfish, one by one, cleaning them off, and throwing them back into the ocean.

As he reached the young girl, the businessman said, "Little girl, I couldn't help but notice what you were doing as I walked toward you. I'm sorry to tell you this, but what you're doing can't possibly make any difference. I have been watching you for the last 15 minutes as I walked along," he said, "and you've only been able to clear this one small little area about 7 feet around." He continued, "There are thousands of starfish on this beach and maybe millions more that we can't even see," he said, sweeping his arm back to the right. "So, I'm sorry to tell you this, but what you're doing can't possibly make any difference."

Looking down at the starfish in her hand, the little girl said, "It does to *this* one!" as she threw the starfish back into the sea.

Well, as I said, it's a hokey story, and I'm not sure it even happened.

But that's what *you* do—isn't it? Every time you take care of a patient, every time you come to work, every time you help out one of your colleagues, you make a difference in people's lives.

If you have children, ask them what they want to do with their lives, and they'll tell you the same thing that our children told us—"I want to make a difference in people's lives!" There is a word for people who work hard for others, who strive valiantly, sometimes against what seem like impossible odds, and all for the good of others.

Do you know what the word is? It's *hero*.

Here's our question to you. When you work here at our hospital and healthcare system, do you feel like a hero? You should! Because if you're not a hero, who is? You take care of those who can't, won't, or don't understand how to take care of themselves. You do it person by person, day by day, week by week, year in and year out. You do it with style, grace, dignity, and equanimity. You are a hero. You are a star thrower!

In many respects, the sum of the message of moments of truth is contained in that story. We have told it to thousands of people at hundreds of hospitals, all with dramatic effect. We invite you to do the same. At our institution, all of our new hires hear the star thrower story. Appropriately enough, our employees of the month and of the quarter are known as the Stars of the ER. They receive, along with their gift certificates and gift cards, a framed certificate with a logo—a starfish.

Whether you use this story or another, it's important that you find a way to help your staff understand not only that they make a difference in people's lives but also that they are heroes. This is the essence of any successful service excellence program—helping the A-Team recognize the heroism of their work—playing a part in serving others in the time of their deepest need, when their health or that of their family and loved ones is at stake. Our fondest hope is that the three Survival

Skills presented in this and the preceding two chapters—making the customer service diagnosis, as well as the technical diagnosis, and offering the right treatment; negotiating for agreement and resolution expectations; and creating moments of truth—will, when combined, help you achieve two goals for you and your staff:

Goal 1—To make the job easier (the real reason to develop a service excellence initiative)

Goal 2—To help you and your staff realize anew that you are engaged in one of the world's most honored professions: giving care and comfort to those who entrust their lives and health to us

In closing, we turn to the words of a truly great human being, Albert Schweitzer, MD (1998):

Of all the will toward the ideal in mankind, only a small part can manifest itself in public action. All the rest of this force must be content with small and obscure deeds. The sum of these, however, is a thousand times stronger than the acts of those who receive wild public recognition. The latter, compared to the former, are like the foam on the waves of a deep ocean.

We gain great satisfaction from teaching service excellence to our colleagues in healthcare across this great nation. But as we travel and come to know people like you and your staff, we realize how true Dr. Schweitzer's words are—we are like the foam on the deep ocean of the good works that you and your staff do. Our hope is that our work makes your work a little easier.

SURVIVAL SKILLS SUMMARY

◆ Your staff constantly create moments of truth for patients thousands of times a day—the sum of which creates the reputation of your healthcare system.
◆ The third Survival Skill is *creating moments of truth*.
◆ From the customer's perspective, the people performing the service *are* the company.
◆ Better to have one person practicing empowered customer service than a hundred posted mission statements proclaiming it.
◆ It's not the mission statement, it's your staff in action that creates service in the organization.

- Service excellence is never complete—it has to be gained every day, in every patient encounter.
- As the leader, round regularly and visibly on patients' units.
- Solve service problems—on the spot.
- Patient care unit directors should greet every admitted patient and give him or her their card, a smile, and the reassurance that "I'm here to help if you need me."
- Hire right—screen for the customer service gene.
- Use your surveys as a tool, not a club.
- Patient satisfaction surveys are an open-book test.
- Use the open-book test approach—huddle up.
  - Analyze each question for A-Team and B-Team behaviors.
  - Recognize the power of scripts.
  - Develop scripts to accentuate A-Team behaviors toward achieving service excellence.
- Celebrate success—create service legends.
- Tell the star thrower (or a similar) story to help your staff understand that what they do is heroic—and that they are, in fact, heroes.

REFERENCES

Carlzon, J. 1987. *Moments of Truth: New Strategies for Today's Customer-Driven Economy*. New York: HarperCollins.

Centers for Medicare & Medicaid Services (CMS). 2013. "HCAHPS: Patients' Perspectives of Care Survey." Washington, DC: CMS.

Eiseley, L. 1978. "The Star Thrower." In *The Star Thrower*, 169–85. Fort Washington, PA: Harvest Books.

Greenleaf, R. K. 2002. *Servant Leadership: A Journey into the Nature of Legitimate Power and Greatness*. New York: Paulist Press.

Peters, T. 2010. *The Little Big Things: 163 Ways to Pursue Excellence*. New York: Harper Business.

Robinson, B. C., K. Cook, and Q. Studer. 2010. *The HCAHPS Handbook: Hardwire Your Hospital for Pay-for-Performance Success*. Pensacola, FL: Firestarter Press.

Sanders, B. 1995. *Fabled Service: Ordinary Acts, Extraordinary Outcomes*. San Diego: Pfieffer.

Schweitzer, A. 1998. *Out of My Life and Work*. Baltimore, MD: John Hopkins University Press.

Spector, R., and P. McCarthy. 1995. *The Nordstrom Way*. New York: Wiley.

MORE RESOURCES ON MOMENTS OF TRUTH

Block, P. 2002. *The Answer to How Is Yes*. San Francisco: Berrett-Koehler.

A truly inspirational book from one of the most incisive minds writing about leadership.

Connellan, T. 1997. *Inside the Magic Kingdom: Seven Keys to Disney's Success*. Austin, TX: Bard Press.

A brief book with insights from a service industry leader.

Kotter, J. P. 1996. *Leading Change*. Boston: Harvard Business School Press.

The definitive text on change management, an essential tool for any service excellence initiative.

Press, I. 2002. *Patient Satisfaction: Defining, Measuring, and Improving the Experience of Care*. Chicago: Health Administration Press.

A scholarly and detailed approach from the nation's éminence grise in patient satisfaction surveys—and a great friend.

APPENDIX 6.1: SELECT QUESTIONS FROM THE HCAHPS SURVEY

How often did nurses communicate well with patients?
During this hospital stay . . .

◆ how often did nurses treat you with courtesy and respect? (Question 1)
◆ how often did nurses listen carefully to you? (Question 2)
◆ how often did nurses explain things in a way you could understand? (Question 3)

How often did doctors communicate well with patients?
During this hospital stay . . .
+ how often did doctors treat you with courtesy and respect? (Question 5)
+ how often did doctors listen carefully to you? (Question 6)
+ how often did doctors explain things in a way you could understand? (Question 7)

How often did patients receive help quickly from hospital staff?
During this hospital stay . . .
+ after you pressed the call button, how often did you get help as soon as you wanted it? (Question 4)
+ how often did you get help in getting to the bathroom or in using a bedpan as soon as you wanted? (Question 11)

How often was patients' pain well controlled?
During this hospital stay . . .
+ how often was your pain well controlled? (Question 13)
+ how often did the hospital staff do everything they could to help you with your pain? (Question 14)

How often did staff explain about medicines before giving them to patients?
Before giving you any new medicine . . .
+ how often did hospital staff tell you what the medicine was for? (Question 16)
+ how often did hospital staff describe possible side effects in a way you could understand? (Question 17)

How often were patients' rooms and bathrooms kept clean?
During this hospital stay . . .
+ how often were your room and bathroom kept clean? (Question 8)

How often was the area around patients' rooms quiet at night?
During this hospital stay . . .
+ how often was the area around your room quiet at night? (Question 9)

Were patients given information about what to do during their recovery at home?
During this hospital stay . . .
+ did hospital staff talk with you about whether you would have the help you needed when you left the hospital? (Question 19)

◆ did you get information in writing about what symptoms or health problems to look out for after you left the hospital? (Question 20)

How do patients rate the hospital?
◆ Using any number from 0 to 10, where 0 is the worst hospital possible and 10 is the best hospital possible, what number would you use to rate this hospital during your stay? (Question 21)

Would patients recommend the hospital to friends and family?
◆ Would you recommend this hospital to your friends and family? (Question 22)

Source: Excerpted from the 2013 HCAHPS survey (CMS 2013).

Part III

THE A-TEAM TOOL KIT

CHAPTER 7

The A-Team Tool Kit,
and the Three Key A-Team Behaviors

We have framed this leadership for great customer service discussion by establishing the following concepts:

- The primary "why" of customer service is that it makes your job easier.
- The A-Team and B-Team exercise is a key step in gaining service excellence.
- Understanding patient expectations is a hallmark of top-performing organizations.
- Achieving patient loyalty—by exceeding patients' and families' expectations—drives your journey toward success.
- Are they patients, or are they customers? They are always both, to varying degrees.
- The more horizontal they are, the more they are patients. The more vertical they are, the more they are customers.
- The first Survival Skill is to make the customer service diagnosis and offer the right treatment.
- The second Survival Skill is to negotiate agreement on and resolution of expectations.
- The third Survival Skill is to create moments of truth in the clinical encounter.

So we've moved through the "why" and introduced the "how" in achieving great customer service. Now it's time to dive into the specifics of the "how."

Chapters 8 through 17 explore ten proven strategies that come from the trenches of our work with more than 200 hospitals and healthcare systems. They are listed in a specific order, but none is more important than any others, as they are, we think you will see, interrelated in very important ways. Each of them provides a highly evidenced-based, tested way to—you guessed it—*make the job easier.* We call this a mantra, because it is a verbal talisman of sorts, repeated as often as necessary to keep the focus where it should be. As an old adage goes, "The main thing is to make sure the main thing stays the main thing."

The main thing here, then, is to make sure that the focus is on keeping the focus trained on the real focus—making the job easier. The three A-Team behaviors and the entire A-Team Tool Kit train a laser-like focus on that goal. They do so by operating under the mind-set that *service is a discipline* and not some rah-rah message to exhort the troops.

The behaviors and tools of the A-Team are built on Aristotle's ancient wisdom from the *Nicomachean Ethics* (Aristotle [350 B.C.] 1999):

We are what we repeatedly do. Excellence, then, is not a virtue, but a habit.

What better way to illustrate that it is discipline, not just abstract commitment to service, that is necessary to motivate people? Another way to characterize the concept is as a "bias towards action" (Peters and Waterman 1982). A culture that is embodied on paper is distinctly different than a culture embodied in disciplined, daily action that is emblematic of that culture.

THE THREE A-TEAM BEHAVIORS

With that central tenet in mind, the remainder of the book is focused on *how* to put evidence-based behaviors and specific tools in the hands of those charged with the difficult task of offering the best possible care through the highest clinical and service quality in the most safe and reliable fashion. In this chapter, we present the three A-Team behaviors that reinforce the A-Team Tool Kit:

1. Sitting down and using open body language
2. Becoming an active listener
3. Practicing effective apology making and blameless apology making

Sitting Down

While it may seem obvious, we have found that staff often benefit from reminders that taking the time to sit down in every clinical encounter with the patient and family is one of the most powerful and important actions they can take. It is odd in the extreme that we are not teaching this behavior to all of our staff—especially the doctors and nurses—because it meets several critical goals:

- It invests time—arguably everyone's most valuable asset—in ways that expand the perception of the limited time we have.
- It changes the entire power/control vector by putting us at eye level with our patients.
- It allows us to use open body language (discussed separately in the next section), which improves communication further.

Sitting down is a discrete and largely unexpected act that shows the provider is taking the time to *move to the patient's level*. Does it take more time than simply standing? Let's assume for the moment that it actually does take more time. (Obviously, we disagree with this postulate, but we'll come back to that.) There is a huge difference between *taking time* and *investing time*. B-Team members often say, "I don't have time for this patient satisfaction nonsense—I'm far too busy for that!" That's an example of someone who views service excellence as taking time from his very busy day. A-Team members view sitting down (as well as the other evidence-based skills of customer service) as an investment of time in that they are wisely using the time they have to gain the maximum payoff. They are leveraging the use of their time in ways that work best, both for them and for the patients. Furthermore, they are investing time in the *relationship* with the patients and their families, as opposed to simply exchanging information.

For example, numerous studies from multiple areas of the healthcare field have shown that when asked, patients and families estimate that the physician or nurse who sits during the visit is present in the room three to five times longer than the clinician who stands (Mayer and Jensen 2009; Groopman 2007; Strauss and Mayer 2014). Further, recent studies from our group (Mayer et al. 2014) indicate that patients rate the quality of the interaction much higher—and thus the patient loyalty ratings are much higher—when the caregiver sits. That's quite a return on investment, or ROI.

When combined with scripts, the sitting down behavior can result in powerful relationship building, as suggested by these examples:

Emergency physician to emergency department (ED) patient: "Mrs. Smith, I am Dr. Cates, the emergency physician who will be taking care of you today. I'm sorry you're not feeling well, but I'm happy to be here to help. I've read your nurses' notes, but let me sit here so we can chat and make sure I understand what's been going on."

Anesthesiologist to patient during preoperative visit: "Mr. Jones, I'm Dr. Hicks, and I am going to be making sure we take care of your anesthesia and pain management during your surgery and in the post-op period. I'd like to sit and spend a few minutes with you to make sure we have all the information we need to make this a safe and even enjoyable experience."

It is critically important when we have the difficult task of breaking bad news to patients and families that we not only sit down but also establish physical contact prior to sharing information about their health. There is, and has always been, a magic to the physical touch of physicians and nurses, and none more important than when we have to tell patients news that, by nature, is difficult to hear. Following is one example:

Hospitalist to a patient who has had a PET scan: (Sits in a chair pulled next to the bed, establishes eye contact, and gently puts her hand in the patient's.) "Mr. Ambrose, I've just gone over your chest scan with the radiologist. I'm afraid that shadow we saw on the X-ray is a tumor. I know that's hard news to hear. The team taking care of you feels the next step is to do a bronchoscopy so we can get some tissue to find out exactly what we are dealing with. Again, I'm sorry to break this result to you, but I wanted to tell you myself and let you know as soon as possible."

Sitting down represents a meaningful time investment not only for physicians but for nurses and other members of the healthcare team as well. The radiology technicians in our ED, for example, are taught to sit down and explain to patients what studies will be done and to ask them if they have any questions. Not surprisingly, they get extremely high patient satisfaction scores.

But what if your clinical staff have no *means* to sit and talk with the patient? To sit in a patient's room requires that the room have chairs or stools. Leaders should take a hard look at their facilities to ensure that there is adequate space and a place to sit. (For that matter, outpatient clinics and EDs also need to have hangers for the patients' clothes and a hook on the wall or the back of the door—otherwise, the clothes often end up on a chair or stool.)

Open Body Language

Sitting down also helps promote clinicians' use of *open body language.* If you are standing by the side or at the foot of the bed, crossing your arms across your chest is, frankly, a very comfortable way to stand. Unfortunately, standing with your arms crossed inadvertently sends a "closed" message to the patients and families. It connotes, "I'm closed—you can't come in." This message is not intentional, of course, but it is undeniable, based on decades of research.

The second most common position for a person standing by the bedside is to have her hands in her pockets, particularly for doctors wearing white coats. While this is also a comfortable position, most patients and families interpret this posture as a sign of boredom or impatience.

Sitting down nearly forces you to lean forward instead of backward and makes it very easy to open your arms and even gesture to the patient with your hands while listening and talking. Patients interpret this open body language positively, as long as you do not get excessively close to them and invade their personal space. Nodding appreciatively and saying "Yes" during the history is also very helpful when combined with open body language.

Active Listening

As we mention in Chapter 5, one of the most useful techniques for effective negotiations and resolution of issues is active listening. Active listening helps assure the patient and family that we are engaged in the conversation; equally important, it also helps ensure that the history being taken is accurate and that the patient's understanding of the clinical workup is clear, that she knows where she is in the journey from horizontal to vertical, and that she has a solid grasp of what to expect in the course of her care.

As we define it earlier in the book, active listening is a communication tool in which the listener systematically feeds back what he has heard the speaker say in order to

- ◆ improve clarity of the message,
- ◆ make listening a participative process, and
- ◆ ensure common ground is reached in the ongoing process of communication.

Repeat the Last Word/Phrase

You may have read elsewhere that the listener should rephrase or paraphrase what the speaker has said. We have found that the best initial response to another's statement is to repeat the last word or phrase the speaker used to improve active listening, as demonstrated in the following example:

Repeat the last word or phrase the patient has used . . .
   "And the worst thing is that I was in so much pain."
   "Pain?"
. . . and then listen some more.
   "Yes, it was unbearable, and no one seemed to care."
   "No one seemed to care?"
   "Yes—that's what offended me!"

In this example, the physician's repetition of the patient's last word or phrase helps the patient continue to voice his concerns and leads to a very important final message from this patient: It was not so much the pain that mattered to him as the fact that no one seemed to care. When a manager is feeding back information on how to improve listening and communication, "pain" is a completely different (if related) message from "no one seemed to care."

Employ the 5 Whys

Another important tool for improving the active listening skill was originally described by Frederick Reichheld (1996), of Bain & Company, in his landmark book, *The Loyalty Effect*. It is known as the "5 Whys" because it teaches the listener to ask "Why?" five times before reaching a preliminary conclusion regarding the nature of the problem. Here's an example:

Patient	Healthcare manager
"I was very unhappy with my visit to your ED."	"Why?"
"The quality of care was horrible."	"Why (do you say that)?"
"Communication was completely absent."	"Why (was that the case)?"
"They contacted the wrong doctor."	"Why (was it the wrong doctor)?"
"My insurance doesn't cover that doctor."	"Why (doesn't it)?"
"She doesn't accept my insurance plan anymore."	—

By using the 5 Whys, the administrator has discovered that the issue is not one of care quality but rather has to do with the patient's insurance plan—a dramatically different issue that requires a different follow-up approach.

Use Scripts

Scripts (Chapter 12) are another way to support active listening, by changing the standard listening dynamic to one that is more effective. Here, we're talking about an insight we shared earlier in the book:

When you're ready to talk, they (the patients) are not ready to listen.

(Trust us, if you have adolescent children, that's one you need to write down.)

Think about discharge instructions. At most hospitals and healthcare systems, there is widespread understanding of the importance of discharge instructions. (This understanding is so pervasive that many questionnaires include this question: Were you given, and did you understand, your discharge instructions?) But do clinicians clearly convey that importance to patients?

Say we introduce a script that each clinician uses to promote that message:

Discharge instructions are very important to us. We want to make sure you understand your discharge instructions.

If every doctor and nurse uses that script every time with every patient, do you think your patient satisfaction scores will go up? The answer, of course, is "Yes."

But here's the *far* more important question: Does that mean each patient truly understands the discharge instructions? On reflection, we can probably all agree that the answer is "No."

The reason for this odd dissonance is that, while we think it is sufficient for us to say that discharge instructions are important *to us*, the fact is, the patients aren't truly listening to us.

When you're giving them discharge instructions, they are looking at your tie, thinking, "That's got to be a yard sale tie, doesn't it? There is no way anyone would ever have paid serious money for that tie!" In other words, the patients are involved in *passive listening*—they are simply listening to us and are not actively involved in the conversation.

But you can change the dynamic by changing the script:

Discharge instructions are very important to us. We want to make sure you understand your discharge instructions. *In fact, they are so important to us that I am going to ask you to repeat the discharge instructions back to me when I am done.*

Now, do you think they will understand and be able to repeat the discharge instructions? You bet they will—there's a *test* at the end of the discharge instructions!

Because they have to understand the discharge instructions well enough to articulate them back to the staff, the patient and his family attend to more fully comprehending the discharge instructions themselves. That's the difference between active and passive listening.

Regardless of which specific techniques are used, active listening is a fundamental discipline that all healthcare personnel should use in their daily care of patients.

Effective Apology Making and Blameless Apology Making

Just as most people believe (incorrectly, as we've shown) that *listening* is an innate and natural human skill, they also believe that *apologizing* is an assumed skill. Nothing could be further from the truth. First, we often take for granted the power of apology. In fact, effective apology making is one of the most powerful and liberating things we can do, primarily because of its *healing power*. What could be more important in healthcare? But the healing is not just for the other person; more importantly, through the power of the apology we can heal ourselves.

Marshall Goldsmith says, "I regard apologizing as the most magical, healing, restorative gesture human beings can make" (Goldsmith, Lyons, and McArthur 2012).

Note that this quote doesn't specify that the magic is restricted to those to whom the apology is given. Of course, effective apology making helps heal our relationship with others, but it also helps us heal, both by opening us to the possibility that we will be forgiven and by "closing the energy packet," as our friend Joan Kyes would say. It puts the issue either behind us or, at a minimum, in an appropriate context should the issue be revisited. (As Ben Franklin said, "Your words say you are sorry. Your actions do not." More on that in a moment.)

The problem with apology making is that very few of our parents, teachers, coaches, and mentors ever taught us how to apologize—and those who did often taught us *wrong*. We certainly weren't taught how to do it in medical, nursing, or hospital administration school, although a rich literature is now emerging in patient safety indicating that admitting mistakes to patients and their families not only is an effective risk reduction strategy but also has important effects on future healing.

Like all the other tools and strategies in our work, apology making is a disciplined, evidence-based practice. Done properly, we extend ourselves (not just our words but our*selves*) to others by accepting responsibility in a way that makes clear that we value the relationship enough to freely admit whatever blame or responsibility is attendant to our actions.

It should not focus on who's "right" and who's "wrong" but rather the ongoing relationship. As John Kador (2009) says in his book, *Effective Apology*, "Effective apology is not about the situation that prompted it, but about the relationship that requires it."

In healthcare, our relationships with our patients and with those who care for our patients (remember BestPractices' Rule 1 and Rule 2?) are fundamental—indeed sacred—to our ability to serve them with trust as the cement that holds it all together. Here's a true story that I (TM) experienced in raising three boys who are now accomplished and talented young men:

> I have always been a "morning person," arising early in the day most mornings. My wife is . . . not. So when Josh, Kevin, and Gregory were younger, it was easier for me to get up; work out; get showered, shaved, and dressed; and be ready to make breakfast for the guys before they took off for school. I liked to use this time not just to chat but also to give them a few "Life Lessons from Dad." One morning we were doing just that when my wife, Maureen, awoke earlier than usual and walked into the kitchen just as I was saying to these fine young men, "OK, say it back to me."
>
> They responded, dutifully if somewhat bored, but very much in unison, "I'm sorry . . . I was wrong . . . it will never happen again."
>
> Maureen said, "What are you doing?" To which I responded, "I'm teaching the boys how to say they're sorry."
>
> She looked at their bored faces and said, "But they don't *mean* it!" And I said, "True, but when they do mean it, at least they'll know how to *say* it!"

We think one of the problems with apologizing is that we haven't been taught how to apologize before we have the need to do so. One way to approach this issue is to emphasize the "count 1, 2, 3, 4" method:

1. "Thanks . . ."
2. "I'm sorry."
3. "I was wrong."
4. "It'll never happen again."

This format works well when we are apologizing for incidents or errors that are directly within our control.

In those situations where we are expressing genuine regret for something that has happened but that is not within our control, apologies can be delivered without assigning blame. Here are some simple examples of "blameless" apologies.

> "I'm sorry you felt you waited too long."
>
> "I'm sorry you felt the doctor was rude to you."

"I'm sorry you felt the nurses were distracted."

"I'm sorry you felt that there was inadequate space in the ED."

"I'm so sorry this happened to you."

We believe there are ten simple steps to delivering an effective apology in healthcare, which are listed below. In the paragraphs that follow, we address the first two on the list.

1. No "ifs," "ands," or "buts."
2. Always use the active voice and short words.
3. Focus on expectations.
4. Don't assume—no "I understand . . ." phrases.
5. "What can I do to make this right?"
6. It's a dialogue, not a monologue.
7. Always begin with "I."
8. Use the person's name.
9. The apology should be tight, staccato-like language; be focused; and have been practiced.
10. Don't argue—the individual is already honked off.

First, as our parents always said, "No 'ifs,' 'ands,' or 'buts'!" Experience with apologies often heard in healthcare actually shows that our "I'm sorries" often sound more like "I have to apologize but I'm not really sorry." Here's a list of actual "apologies" we have heard over the years, followed by a more effective way of dealing with the issue.

Actual Apology	Effective Apology
I'm sorry if what you said is true.	I'm sorry this happened.
I'm sorry if I offended you.	I am so sorry I offended you.
If we were out of line, I am sorry.	We were out of line—I'm sorry.
I'm sorry [and] we have a lot of sicker patients.	I'm sorry. Every patient's needs are important to us.
I'm sorry [and] it's a tough place to work.	I'm sorry. I will address this with the team who cared for you.
I'm sorry, but we can't find good help.	I'm sorry—we lost track of our priorities.
I'm sorry, but you started it!	I'm sorry—this is my fault entirely.

There is also an understandable, if misguided, tendency in healthcare to use long words or arcane phrases and acronyms in passive-voice sentences. Great communicators know that we are always better off in the active voice, with short, staccato language. The list below shows more actual "apologies" we have heard from our experience—all from well-meaning folks whose language and syntax mangled the meaning and intent.

Passive	Active
I'm sorry if therapeutic misadventures were allowed to happen.	I'm sorry we made mistakes.
I'm sorry your medical record was misplaced by inadvertent actions.	I'm sorry we lost your chart.
I'm sorry you were allowed to misinterpret what we were communicating.	I'm sorry we didn't speak more clearly.
I'm sorry the delay in your care was extended longer than we would have liked.	I'm sorry you waited so long.

Effective apology making and blameless apology making don't just happen—they have to be taught, and they have to be practiced. Make sure your orientation, in-service programs, and management team meetings emphasize both how to do it right and how it is often done wrong. We return to the use of effective apologies in the next chapter when we discuss their importance in service recovery.

SURVIVAL SKILLS SUMMARY

- The A-Team Tool Kit puts evidence-based tools in your hands to effectively move from the "why" to the "how" of service excellence.
- The three A-Team Behaviors that should be used in all patient encounters are (1) sitting down and using open body language, (2) active listening, and (3) effective apology making and blameless apology making.
- Sitting down is a highly leveraged investment of time (one of your most important resources) to gain the maximum service ROI.
- Adding appropriate, healing physical contact to sitting down is extremely effective, particularly when stresses are high and the news is bad.
- Sitting down drives us toward more open, effective body language.

- The skills of active listening include repeating the last word or phrase spoken by the patient, asking her to repeat back what she has just been told, and employing the 5 Whys technique.
- Effective apologies are not accidental—there is a skill to them, which can be taught.
- Use the blameless apology format when appropriate.
- When we have made mistakes, we must own up to them and apologize in clear, succinct ways.
- Apologizing not only attempts to wipe a slate clean but also sets the stage for healing on both sides of the relationship.

REFERENCES

Aristotle. (350 B.C.) 1999. *Nicomachean Ethics*, 2nd ed. Reprint, Cambridge, MA: Hackett.

Goldsmith, M., L. S. Lyons, and S. McArthur. 2012. *Coaching for Leadership: Writings on Leadership from the World's Great Coaches.* San Francisco: Pfeiffer.

Groopman, J. 2007. *How Doctors Think.* Boston: Houghton Mifflin.

Kador, J. 2009. *Effective Apology: Mending Fences, Building Trust.* San Francisco: Berrett-Koehler.

Mayer, T., and K. Jensen. 2009. *Hardwiring Flow: Systems and Processes for Seamless Patient Care.* Gulf Breeze, FL: Fire Starter Press.

Mayer, T. A., J. Kaplan, R. W. Strauss, and R. J. Cates. 2014. "Customer Service in Emergency Medicine." In *Strauss and Mayer's Emergency Department Management*, edited by R. W. Strauss and T. A. Mayer. New York: McGraw-Hill.

Peters, T. J., and R. H. Waterman Jr. 1982. *In Search of Excellence: Lessons from America's Best-Run Companies.* New York: Harper Business.

Reichheld, F. F. 1996. *The Loyalty Effect: The Hidden Force Behind Growth, Profits, and Lasting Value.* Boston: Harvard Business Press.

Strauss, R. W., and T. A. Mayer. 2014. "Scripts: Using Evidence-Based Language to Improve Service." In *Strauss and Mayer's Emergency Department Management*, edited by R. W. Strauss and T. A. Mayer. New York: McGraw-Hill.

MORE RESOURCES ON THE A-TEAM AND ACTIVE LISTENING

Hoppe, M. 2006. *Active Listening: Improving Your Ability to Listen and Lead.* Greensboro, NC: Center for Creative Leadership.

Shafir, R. Z. 2003. *The Zen of Listening.* Wheaton, IL: Quest Books.

These are two succinct books on active listening.

CHAPTER 8

A-Team Tool 1—Empowerment: Point-of-Impact Intervention, Service Recovery, Leading Up

Empowerment. Great word. Great concept. Yet often overused and misunderstood. Motivational speaker Tom Peters calls empowerment "purposeful chaos" and "the great energy liberator" (Peters and Waterman 2004). But what does it have to do with service excellence?

Empowerment is the sustained and deep commitment to a philosophy that well-selected, well-trained staffs are our most important resource and they deserve to have the authority to make appropriate decisions over the span of influence for which they are held accountable. To empower your staff, simply enact a policy today that states, *Make no decisions at a higher level that can be made at a lower level.*

As we've stated repeatedly, healthcare is a personal service business. The unit of transaction is always a person. It's not a chest X-ray or a coronary artery stent or a bronchoscopy or a laparoscopic cholecystectomy. It's all of these—and many more—done *by* people *for* patients. As we mention in Chapter 6, the third Survival Skill is to create moments of truth in the clinical encounter, the most immediate and important corollary of which is that the people who deliver the service have enormous power to shape patients' perceptions of the healthcare system.

A policy of empowerment takes this concept a step further by making clear that the people responsible for service delivery must be entrusted with the power to provide meaningful service. That doesn't mean that appropriate checks and supervision aren't in place; it means that staff should be able to make their own decisions when appropriate. Too often in healthcare, however, we are told that when it comes to empowerment, the words and the music don't match.

At one prestigious medical center with a reputation for having empowerment programs, we asked a large audience of employees a simple question: "Are you empowered?" The silence was, frankly, a bit uncomfortable, until a small voice from the last row said, "They *tell* us we are." You tell your staff they are empowered, but where's the substance of the empowerment, and how do you give it to them? Often in healthcare, the words (*empowerment*) and the music (*empowerment in action*) don't match.

THICK-RULEBOOK ORGANIZATIONS VERSUS THIN-RULEBOOK ORGANIZATIONS

Healthcare organizations that deliver true service excellence understand that service doesn't reside in a customer service manual, in a service department, or in a thick rulebook that explains every detail of how to act, how to dress, what to say, what to do, what not to do. In fact, organizations that have thick service rulebooks often deliver robot-like service. We've all experienced the B-Team employee who says, voice dripping with sarcasm:

"Of *course* I care. Your happiness is *very* important to me."

We actually had one person who at least had the candor to tell us:

"You can make me *say* this stuff—but you can't make me *mean* it!"

Greatness in service comes from thin rulebooks, not thick ones. Thick-rulebook organizations delineate everything about how, and every way in which, service is to be delivered and insist on adherence. Thin-rulebook organizations create the broad and important mission and vision regarding service and the organizations' commitment to it, but they rely on leadership and management to act as catalysts to help employees discover, uncover, and create service excellence in ways that they know better than you ever could. It is wise to remember that it is *better to have one person practicing empowered customer service than a hundred posted mission statements proclaiming it.*

Make your commitment to service excellence clear, but keep a thin rulebook—then turn your staff loose to create that level of service. Celebrate service success stories and reward your champions (Chapter 16), and A-team behaviors (invented by them, not you) will flourish.

NARROW CORRIDORS FOR SUCCESS, OR WIDE CORRIDORS FOR SUCCESS?

Service excellence occurs in organizations that have not only thin rulebooks but also wide corridors for success. There are many ways in which to succeed in service—not just "the boss's way" or "the company's way." If your organization is one in which you hear the familiar quote, "My way or the highway," you can be certain that neither empowerment nor service excellence will occur. These organizations have narrow corridors for success in that there are specific, tightly defined pathways that *must* be followed. The better alternative is to have wide corridors for success by hiring right (as we discuss in Chapter 13), training staff well, giving them servant leaders who exemplify the service ethic, and then turning them loose. They will create more great service than a leadership team could possibly imagine, as the rest of the chapter illustrates. Trying to narrow people's options for success is less effective than establishing a clear vision and affording them the creativity to widen the ways in which they can succeed.

THE EMPOWERMENT PARADOX: EMPOWERED ACCOUNTABILITY

Experienced and astute leaders have overcome the fundamental paradox of making no decisions at a higher level that can be made at a lower level while doing so in an evidence-based, disciplined culture of accountability. On the one hand, we say, "Do whatever is necessary for the good of the patient . . ." and on the other hand, it's ". . . and here are the tools with which to do it." Practicing a philosophy of empowered accountability certainly points to a dynamic tension, but one that we find both resolvable and, frankly, typical of most effective change initiatives. After all, the rulebook may be *thin*, but there *is* a rulebook. The corridors may be wide, but there *are* corridors.

Empowerment should always be guided by M/V/V—the mission, vision, and values of the organization—but particularly the values, which should reflect the core and largely unchanging beliefs of the organization. We aren't asking our team to "just wing it" but rather empowering them with both the wisdom of our organizational values and the framework of evidence-based experience.

As healthcare leaders, we aspire to attain positions from which we can influence others to do great things. What we forget is that we are *always* in a position, regardless of our level in the organization or our span of responsibility, to influence others, often in ways we could scarcely have imagined until we recognized the results of our impact. When we lead our lives in ways that reflect core values, we encourage others by example to do the same—to *em-power* those values by putting them into action.

Committing to empowerment—and to the thoughtfulness, kindness, and appreciation that underpin it—doesn't mean we won't hold staff accountable. It *does* mean that we will give them every available resource, every possible opportunity, and the widest berth possible to do the right things for patients and their loved ones.

In thinking about how to deliver the message of empowerment, remember the advice variously attributed to Plato, Philo of Alexandria, and Ian Maclaren (the pseudonym of Rev. John Watson):

Be kind, because everyone you meet is fighting a great battle.

The work we do in the service of healing is never easy—anyone who thinks it is has probably never done it. But we "fight the great battle" for others, not for ourselves, as the "Starfish" story in Chapter 6 is meant to illustrate. Our patients are also fighting the great battle back to health as they undertake their journey from horizontal to vertical, as we discuss in Chapter 3. The kindness we show in our daily work should be reflected in the empowerment of our entire team, *and that empowerment should be directed not just to patients but to our team members as well.*

Here's a story from one of us (TM) that reflects the importance of those who might seem to have the least power but in fact have a tremendous impact on the lives of others.

I was a theology major, and a football player as well—not exactly what you might expect of someone who ended up going to medical school. As it turned out, I had taken a course in biology just to meet a science requirement. My professor, Dr. Enos Pray, saw something in me. He pulled me aside one day and said, "Thom, have you thought about the idea that you might actually have more impact on people's lives as a physician than as a theologian?" That began a journey that saw me taking all the requirements for medical school in a very short period of time. Many of those courses were in chemistry.

In my first chemistry course, I was pretty much lost. I was taking the midterm exam, and I was certain that it wasn't going well at all. At the end of the test, there was an envelope marked "Bonus Question." I opened the envelope and found a piece of paper that said, "If you get this question correct, you will get an 'A' on this test, no matter what you have scored on the rest of the test." I unfolded the page and it read, "What is the name of the man who cleans this room every night so you can have a great environment in which to learn?" Smiling, I walked up to Professor Keith White, the chair of the Chemistry Department and the man who taught the course.

"Uh, Dr. White, on the bonus question, do you want the first name or the last name?" I asked. He paused and then said, "Son, if you can give me the first name *and* the last name, I will not only give you an 'A' on this test, I will give you an 'A' for the entire course!"

Not quite content, I asked, "What if I can give you the names and ages of all of his kids?"

Dr. White was clearly stunned. He took off his glasses and said, very seriously, "Thom, if you can do that, I will give you an 'A' in every course you take from me—so long as you do your best in each of them."

I returned to my desk, wrote out the names and ages of the janitor and his children—and threw in his wife's name for extra measure. Dr. White was as good as his word, and I ended up with a major in chemistry as well.

True story. I give Dr. White all the credit for having the wisdom to ask that question, particularly of a room filled with ambitious pre-med majors competing for grades. He was telling us, of course, that some things are more important—much more important—than chemical reactions and equations. It is always about people.

By the way, the reason that I knew the janitor and his family is that I did a lot of my work in the chemistry lab late at night, after football practice and classes were over. I had a lot of ground to make up. The janitor always said the same thing: "Burning the midnight oil again. Someone has a fire in his belly!" But here's the key—I didn't befriend the janitor; he befriended me. His name was Roosevelt Jones, and I will never forget him.

The transformational leader Martin Luther King Jr. said in his sermon "The Three Dimensions of Life," delivered April 9, 1967, at the New Covenant Baptist Church in Chicago:

> If a man is called to be a street sweeper, he should sweep streets even as Michelangelo painted, or Beethoven composed music, or Shakespeare wrote poetry and plays. He should sweep streets so well that all the hosts of heaven and earth will pause to say, "Here lived a great street sweeper, who did his job well and joyfully." (King 1967)

As we note in Chapter 1, each person has to discover where his deep joy intersects the world's deep needs. We can't operate our healthcare systems without people at every level of life, each of whom is necessary to our success and without whom we couldn't even open our doors.

So, empower your staff to deliver not just for their patients but for their team as well.

Try this exercise. Write the following words on the board at a staff meeting:

Do the best you can.

Ask a member of your staff to read it. Ask another . . . and another . . . and another . . . and still another. Pay a great deal of attention to how they say it. Where is the *emphasis*? And what is the *punctuation and inflection* they give to it? It will seem strange, both to them and perhaps to you at first, but there is an important point to this exercise.

Many will put the emphasis on "best," others on "do," and still others on "can." Very, very few will put the emphasis on "you." So what? We suggest that not only do words matter but the arrangement and emphasis of those words matter. Behaviors matter. The sequence and context of those behaviors matter more. Here's a summary of our experience with what the emphasis on those different words means to those who say them.

Do the best you can.

Emphasis	Meaning
"best"	Focus on excellence, but often extrinsically motivated
"Do"	Focus on action: Do something, even if it's wrong
"can"	Focus on execution, what's possible
"you"	Focus on the individual: What can *you* do?

There are no right or wrong answers here, but we gently suggest that those who put the emphasis on *you* probably understand the wisdom that we should always be kind "because everyone you meet is fighting a great battle." We are all doing the best *we* can.

With that in mind, we turn to the three A-Team empowerment tools.

EMPOWERMENT: POINT-OF-IMPACT INTERVENTION

After studying patients' complaints and concerns carefully for more than 20 years, we uncovered an important fact: More than 95 percent of the time medical errors occur, the caregiver realizes there is a problem or potential problem *at the time the patient's care is delivered.*

Point-of-Impact Skills

For that reason, we created the point-of-impact intervention model. It represents the intersection of two vectors—empowerment and negotiation skills—to make clear to our staff that they are empowered to solve problems when they occur using negotiation skills. Point-of-impact intervention involves the following eight steps.

1. Identify the problem and address it immediately.
Whoever identifies the problem should let the patient know that they are aware something has gone wrong and that they want to "fix it." They should convey that they understand that the patient's expectations have not been met.

2. Establish the fact that you know there has been a breakdown.
Use the two most powerful words in the English language: *I'm sorry.* Say it early, and say it often. Make sure it is used liberally. Add the blameless apology, as described in Chapter 7, to acknowledge the fact that some service standard has been breached, that you apologize for it, but that you do so in a blameless way. For example:

> "I'm sorry it's taken so long to see you, but I'll try to move you through the system as fast as possible from this point on."

It *doesn't* say, "I'm sorry we're turkeys" or "I'm sorry everyone *else* is a turkey" or even "I'm sorry you had to wait, but we couldn't give a flip what time you get seen." It's a sincere apology, but it does not assess blame, as assessing blame at the time of the complaint is usually a waste of time, effort, and energy.

Another example:

> "I'm sorry you felt the staff were rude."

Did you just say the staff were rude? No—simply that you are sorry the patient *felt* the staff were rude. Big difference.

3. Wipe the slate clean.

Try to get to the proverbial tabula rasa. Use phrases such as, "I know you feel this hasn't gone well up to this point, but let me see if I can help you through this." Here's a story Dr. Sharon Day, one of our pediatric emergency physicians, told us:

> I was coming on the morning shift and was on sign-out rounds with the night doctor, who was explaining to me that because they had lost the spinal fluid sample on a child for whom they were ruling out meningitis, they had to redo the spinal tap. I saw the father sitting in the room, obviously frustrated, angry, and extremely tired from a long night—and with his child getting not one but two spinal taps. I thought to myself, "We are going to get a seriously angry letter from this guy!" But I put my arm on the father's shoulder and said, "Sir, I know you've had a long night, and you look really tired. Can I get you a cup of coffee? I'll make sure your son's care goes as fast as it possibly can from this point forward." He took the coffee—and we did get a letter. However, it was a letter of compliment, not complaint.

With that one simple act, she wiped a tarnished slate clean—and created great service. That's a "two-fer": She not only killed a complaint but generated a compliment.

4. Reestablish their expectations.

Our studies (Mayer and Cates 1999; Mayer et al. 1998) indicate that more than 90 percent of patients' complaints arise from an initial failure to clearly establish the patient's or family's expectations. In essence, the wrong customer service diagnosis is made and is therefore being treated incorrectly. Reestablish or clarify their expectations, and *then* treat the *right* customer service diagnosis.

5. Negotiate and resolve issues.

Give your staff the power and authority to solve issues on the spot. Can they give out meal tickets, offer coffee bar courtesies, or write off bills? One system in Michigan hands out movie tickets if the patient waits too long.

6. When possible, meet patients' expectations.

Talk to the patient, relieve his pain, answer his questions. Give him specific time frames for follow-up, and use expectation creation to offer clearly identified expectations, including timelines, of what and when things will happen.

7. Offer reasonable alternatives.

The customer is *not* always right. Nor are the corollary statements "The customer is not always right, but they are always the customer" or "The customer is not always right, but you have to make them think they're right." Don't say such nonsense to your staff. Why? Because if the customer is always right, what does that make you? Always wrong! The point is, you can't always meet every expectation, but you can give patients and families reasonable alternatives using language with a strong service orientation. For example, for patients with chronic pain, it is often not the right thing to do to simply give them more pain medications, but offering to refer them to the hospital's pain management service is an effective alternative, particularly if the team member personally calls and makes the referral, perhaps getting an expedited appointment to personalize the service.

8. When all else fails, give the patient someone else to talk to.

Give your staff the ability to defer to leadership and management's strong service commitment. Let them talk to the charge physician, the charge nurse, or the department director. Give them scripts that say to the patient, "I'm sorry I haven't been able to resolve all of your concerns and expectations. But service is very important to us here. With your permission, I'll leave a voice mail with my manager, and she'll contact you as soon as her schedule allows."

Let staff use the voice mail system to communicate these concerns, and then ensure that leaders and managers are returning calls—preferably within 24 hours.

> Service success requires all leaders and managers, including administrators and CEOs, to be close to the action in service delivery and service recovery.

You say your managers don't have time to field these calls? Then you don't have much of a service excellence program. Service success requires all leaders and managers, including administrators and CEOs, to be close to the action in service delivery and service recovery. When you return these calls, use service recovery skills, as discussed next.

EMPOWERMENT: SERVICE RECOVERY

While point-of-impact intervention is a form of complaint *prevention,* service recovery is a form of complaint *management.* Many hospitals have their own specific system or mnemonic for service recovery; see the "More Resources on Empowerment" section at the end of the chapter for sources that list some of the devices used. Here we give you the mini version:

In person . . .
By phone . . .
By letter . . .
The sooner, the better!

In other words, *how* you contact patients is less important than *how soon* you contact them. The service literature is replete with studies showing that if you identify and resolve a customer's problem within 48 hours of its occurrence, you can retain that customer or even turn him into a loyal customer. As shown in Exhibit 8.1, time is of the essence in service recovery.

Specifically, the exhibit shows that a paradox exists in service recovery: If we are able to recognize when and how we have failed to meet the patient's expectations and then act quickly to address the situation, the patient's loyalty level may actually *rise above* where it had been prior to the service failure.

But if your service recovery exceeds 72 hours, you have likely lost any reasonable chance of recovering that patient's business. Worse yet, some patients become

Exhibit 8.1: Service Recovery Paradox

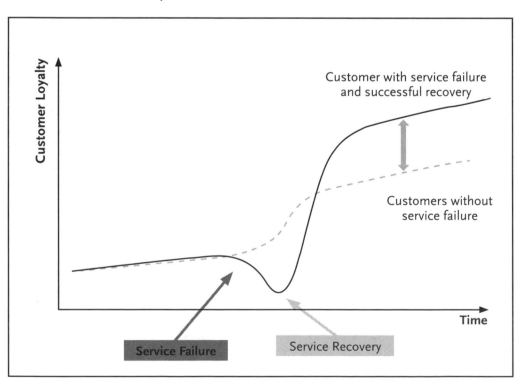

"crusaders," who bad-mouth your healthcare system at every opportunity—to the community, to their friends and neighbors, in public forums, to your board members, even to the press. Transform crusaders using the preventive skills of point-of-impact intervention. If this approach fails, then use the following service recovery skills:

◆ Listen
◆ Apologize
◆ Follow through
◆ Follow up
◆ Offer something extra

Listen

As we've discussed before, of all the communication skills, listening is by far the most important, particularly when a patient/customer feels that her expectations have not been met. Most of this listening will be done on the telephone, although some patients and their families will want to come to your office to talk. For the telephone complaints, get a cup of coffee (and in some cases one of those tall, frothy, foamy drinks) and get comfortable—because you are going to be listening for a *long* time to some complaints.

Like a child with a tantrum, some complainers simply have to wear themselves out. Let them know at the outset that service is important to you and that you would like to know how it can be improved. Take notes and wait until they have had a chance to fully vent their concerns. Use *active listening* to clarify their concerns, employing language such as, "Mrs. Jones, I appreciate your having brought this matter to my attention. Here's what I heard you say regarding your concerns. . . ." Because listening is the most important of all communication skills—and because listening effectively, empathetically, and actively is the most difficult to master—develop it not only in yourself but also in your staff.

Apologize

As we note in more detail in the previous chapter, apologizing is an area that many in healthcare find problematic. Make sure your staff know how to say the two most powerful words in the English language: "I'm sorry." Also as discussed previously, use the blameless apology. You should not be apologizing for your staff, their behavior, the lack of staffing, or other issues. You should let patients/customers know that you're sorry that this problem occurred. The following examples are how *not* to apologize:

- "I'm sorry our staff are morons."
- "I'm sorry the doctor was so obnoxious to you and your family."
- "I'm sorry we are so short staffed."
- "We can't find good help!"

Examples of the blameless apology are the following:

- "I'm sorry this happened to you."
- "I'm sorry you feel that you were ignored."
- "I'm sorry we couldn't do a better job in meeting your expectations."
- "I'm sorry you feel that the staff were rude to you."

The old adage is often true—a gentle word does turn away wrath. Many patients have a genuine and legitimate (in their mind) sense of outrage regarding the complaints they have about their experiences with healthcare. As leaders and managers, it is your job to decompress and decode that outrage in an attempt to turn it into a positive situation, particularly when it comes to using complaints to eliminate B-Team behaviors and to fix your faulty processes.

Fix It

As we indicate in Chapter 1, complaint analysis is one of the most effective tools available to a healthcare leader. Using service failures as a guide toward improving A-Team behaviors; eliminating B-Team behaviors; and empowering staff through feedback, training, and improved processes is essential. Not all complainers are nut cases. As Mark Twain said, "Nothing defines us better than how we behave toward fools." We are certainly not implying that patients who have complaints are fools—far from it. Their insights into how service appears to them can often be gifts that allow you to see yourself and your organization in a light that helps you improve services, processes, and outcomes. But you should pay particular attention when you are handling what you consider to be "unreasonable" expectations.

Not only should you "fix it" in service recovery, you also need to let the patient know that you have used his concerns in a positive fashion as a part of process improvement. A simple statement like, "I appreciate your letting me know about your concerns, as we can only improve our service when people are as kind as you have been in informing us about those concerns" lets the patient know you appreciate his feedback and take his concerns seriously.

Offer Something Extra

Several years ago, I (RJC) handled what at the time seemed to be the "complainer from hell." This gentleman was concerned about the care provided to his daughter (as is often the case, people are usually more distressed about the care provided to their family members than that provided to themselves). He started outraged, stayed outraged, and became more outraged through the course of our attempts at service recovery.

As with many complaints, what set him off had some substance to it—in this case a medical staff member failed to arrive in the emergency department (ED) in a timely fashion and then said something completely unprofessional once he did arrive. The issue was compounded when the medical staff specialist continued to exhibit B-Team behaviors. Although the specialist did not work for us, we understood that whoever identifies the complaint owns the complaint and acts as a guide through the recovery process, including making telephone calls, writing letters, and following up to be sure that the problem has been addressed. To take such an approach, these are the sorts of questions you must ask—and insist that others ask—in your organization:

- Who owns the problem?
- How do you guide the staff back to service success from the patient's perspective?

In this particular case, it seemed as if *nothing* would please this gentleman or turn away his wrath. Multiple phone calls and communications went back and forth over a period of several weeks. (We forgot to mention that he was a lieutenant general—a *three-star* general—in the Marines. Those folks are used to people snapping to attention and following their every order.) Finally, we sent him a letter that read, in part:

> Thank you for taking time from your busy schedule to inform us of your concerns in rich detail, so that we could appropriately address them. Please accept the enclosed gift certificate to Outback Steakhouse as a symbol of our appreciation for the time you took to help us improve our service.

Now, you (or your management team) might say, "There is *no way* that a simple $25 Outback Steakhouse coupon is going to make this problem go away!" But in fact it did—we got a very complimentary letter back from this gentleman, thanking us and indicating that he would certainly use our services if he needed emergency care for his family in the future. We turned a complainer into a loyal customer. Think of it another way: How many doctors do you have on your staff who own both a Jaguar and a Mercedes yet would trample each other to get to the drug representative for a free plastic pen? What do you think they would do to get an Outback Steakhouse coupon?

Everybody loves a gift. Judiciously and appropriately utilized, "something extra" can help put service recovery into a different perspective for the patient. Meal tickets, gift certificates, flowers, fruit baskets—use your imagination, and empower your staff to give such gifts as well.

Clearly, gifts should be restricted to service problems, as opposed to technical problems. If you or your risk management folks believe a patient or family might be litigious, you should avoid offering gifts as a recovery option, as they can be considered offensive or an attempt to "buy off" potential litigants. Notwithstanding such circumstances, for service problems, whether in the form of free meals, free parking, or certificates for the coffee bar in the atrium, gifts can serve as an important part of service recovery.

Follow Through, Follow Up

When a patient takes the time to identify a problem and you agree that, indeed, a behavior, process, or system needs to be fixed, fix it! Assuring patients that you have followed through on their concerns to fix the problem and made sure that it stays fixed is another extremely important part of service recovery—to your staff as well as to the patient. If you are serious about complaint management as a way of improving service recovery and eliminating B-Team behaviors and processes, you must be able to demonstrate that appropriate follow-through has occurred. Once you have evidence that it has taken place, you may reassure the patient/customer of that in your follow-up communications.

EMPOWERMENT: LEADING UP

In the 2008 Beijing Olympic Games, the US men's 4 × 100 track and field relay team not only was expected to win the gold medal but also was likely to set progressive world records in the heats along the way. They were among the best athletes ever assembled, they had clear goals, they were well trained, and they had the highest possible aspirations. Indeed, they had spent their entire athletic lives dreaming of winning an Olympic gold medal. Did they win? They did not.

As inconceivable as it may seem, they dropped the baton. They were great, elite athletes, but they hadn't practiced enough *as a team.* It was assumed that the handoffs would go well after all those years of training, but they hadn't practiced the handoffs together.

How often do we "drop the baton" in healthcare? Unfortunately, far too often.

Healthcare is essentially a series of transitions and handoffs from one team member to another. We continuously pass the baton, even in the simplest of interactions. The following example demonstrates that even a "fast track" patient in the ED with a sprained ankle is likely to encounter numerous people in sequence:

ED greeter: "Hello—can I help you?"

Triage nurse: "What happened?"

Registration: "ID, insurance card, and demographics?"

[Sits in waiting room]

Primary nurse: "Come on back, I'm your nurse. Let's get some ice on that ankle."

Emergency physician: "I'll be taking care of you today. Where does it hurt? Let's have a look. Let's get an X-ray."

Radiology technician: "I'll be taking your film today. Jump up on the table."

Primary nurse: "Let's get the ice back on that ankle. The doctor will be in to see you once she's looked at the X-ray."

Emergency physician: "Good news—there is no fracture. However, you have a second-degree sprain, which hurts as much as a fracture but heals faster. We're going to get a set of crutches and a compressive wrap. Keep the ankle elevated, stay off it for five days, take this medicine for pain, and see your orthopedist in five to seven days for follow-up. Any questions?"

ED technician: "Hi, I'm Augie, the ED tech, and I'm going to get crutches and show you how to use them. How tall are you?"

Primary nurse: "OK, we're all set. Please sign these discharge instructions, and here are your prescriptions, the name of the orthopedic surgeon on call, and a written excuse for missing work."

Even with something as seemingly minor as a sprained ankle, at least ten service transitions take place, where the baton is passed from one person to another. The question is, how effectively are those service transitions being made—or are they essentially left to chance?

We use the term *leading up* to mean that we are passing the baton to the next team member in a way that introduces the patient in a positive light. (Quint Studer calls it "managing up" and defines it as "positioning people well.") Like a world-class relay team, this process has to be practiced and is a part of a discipline, not just a mind-set.

Using the previous example, here are some ways we can lead up across clinical boundaries as we pass the service baton (note that in a leading-up system, time spent in the waiting room is eliminated and the sequence of handoffs changes):

ED greeter: "I'm sorry this happened. Let me get you a wheelchair so you can get off that ankle. I'll wheel you over to triage. Jeff, this is John Jones, and he sprained his ankle playing basketball."

Triage nurse: "Mr. Jones, I'm Jeff, the triage nurse, and I will be getting you started today. We have a set of triage protocols and standing orders for extremity trauma, so let's have look at your foot and ankle to see what X-rays we might need, and then I will get them ordered. We'll put some ice on that and keep your foot elevated to help keep the swelling down. Then registration will take a few minutes to make sure we have your correct contact information. Finally, we'll get you over to Fast Track, which is a special area where we can take care of you more quickly."

Registration: "Hi, Mr. Jones. Jeff let me know that you twisted your ankle. I just need to take a couple of minutes, for your safety and confidentiality, to make sure we have your correct contact information. May I make a copy of your driver's license and any insurance information you might have? Once I'm done, one of the Fast Track nurses will be taking over."

Radiology technician: "Mr. Jones, I'm Tom, the radiology technician, and I'll be taking the films Jeff ordered. Do you have any questions about what we'll be doing?"

Fast Track nurse: "Mr. Jones, I'm Angie, and I will be the nurse caring for you today. I understand that you twisted your ankle playing basketball about an hour ago and that Jeff ordered your X-rays. After I do my assessment, Dr. Fullerton, our Fast Track physician today, will see you. She is terrific, and she'll do a great job for you."

Emergency physician: "Mr. Jones, I'm Dr. Fullerton, and I will be your emergency physician here in Fast Track. I read the notes that Jeff, Angie, and the rest of the team wrote, but let's just recap. After that I'll do a thorough exam and then explain what we see on the X-ray.

[Following exam.] "So my exam and your X-ray findings show this is not a fracture, but it is a second-degree ankle sprain, which hurts just as much as a fracture but, fortunately, heals much faster. I see you've visited Dr. Theiss for orthopedic issues in the past. He's really great, isn't he? My whole family has seen him. You'll need to see him in about five to seven days. In the meantime, we need you to stay off of the ankle, keep it elevated, ice it, and keep a compression bandage on it. We call that "RICE," for rest, ice, compression, and elevate. Augie is our tech in Fast Track today; he's one of the most experienced and best techs we have. He's going to get your crutches, show you how to use them, and put a compression splint on your ankle."

ED technician: "Hi, Mr. Jones. Doc Fullerton asked me to help you—she's a great doc, huh? We love working with her."

On the surface, you might say the technical quality of care is the same in both cases. But is it really? Leading up allows the patient to know much more clearly that we are working as a team, that we know each other and talk with each other, and that we exchange patient information regularly and in a professional and safe manner. This idea returns to a point we have made before: *Technical quality and service quality can never be separated—they are part of one whole patient experience.*

Exhibit 8.2 provides more examples of ways in which we can use leading up to pass the baton effectively to our team members.

You may be thinking, "But what about when we are passing the baton to a B-Team member?" Excellent question, but the answer may seem paradoxical: That is precisely when leading up becomes *most important.* That is when you want to make sure the handoff goes particularly well, and you take the time to let the B-Team members know you have already led them up. Here's an example:

- ◆ "Janet is your nurse today, and she's the best we have."
- ◆ "Let me introduce you to Dr. Smith. He is my partner and will be taking over your care. I have briefed him on everything about your case, and he will take great care of you."
- ◆ "Unfortunately, the bone is broken. The good news is, Dr. Theiss is on call, and he is a great one."
- ◆ "You will need to be admitted. I spoke to your primary care physician, and he wants our specialist in Hospital Medicine to care for you. Dr. Rodriguez will be taking care of you, and she is excellent."

"Hi, Dr. Cranky. I spoke with Mrs. Ramirez and her family and let them know you are the hospitalist who will be taking care of them. I also let them know that we work with you all the time and that you'll do a great job and answer all their questions. Thanks for your help."

All of a sudden, Dr. Cranky starts to live up to the previews you have given the patient and the family. In other words, don't be surprised if leading up starts to move B-Team members to the A-Team.

We close our discussion on leading up with a personal story that clearly illustrates how meaningful this tool can be.

My (TM) father was a World War II veteran, who translated his skills as a tank maintenance expert to a successful auto repair business in my hometown of Anderson, Indiana. His buddies were also WWII vets, and each of them had his own particular business or specialty in the automotive industry. For example, Pop was great at transmission repairs and overhauls, Bob Hobbs ran the best brake service around, his brother Dewey had the wheel alignment business, and Ed Shipley ran the best body shop.

When I would come home from college or medical school, I would always work with Pop, both for the compensation and the camaraderie. I ask people now how many times they think I heard these kinds of statements:

"Hey, Joe College, help me figure out these brakes."

"Hey, Mr. Medical Student, show me how to get this converter back in this transmission."

The answer usually surprises people—*never*. Not once did any of my dad's friends treat me with anything other than complete and total respect.

Years later at Pop's funeral, I told the guys how much it meant to me that they had been so kind to me. All of the guys looked at each other and started laughing. Finally, Dewey Hobbs said, "Thom, your dad gave us strict instructions that we were to treat you with respect. He said, "Don't you give him any grief—he's a good kid!"

That's when I realized Pop had been leading me up before I ever entered the room. You can do the same with your team.

SURVIVAL SKILLS SUMMARY

◆ To empower your team, make no decision at a higher level that can be made at a lower level.

◆ Make sure you have an organization with a thin rulebook and a wide corridor for success.

◆ There is always a paradox between evidence-based empowerment ("Do what needs to be done for the patient") and accountability ("Results matter, and we will measure and account for them").

◆ The rulebook may be thin, but there *is* a rulebook.

◆ Remember this important wisdom: "Be kind, because everyone you meet is fighting a great battle."

◆ Empowerment should be directed not just to dealing with patients and their families but also to dealing with the entire healthcare team.

◆ Help your staff understand the various meanings of "Do the best you can."

◆ Point-of-impact intervention is an evidenced-based approach to ensuring that you have an effective tool in place for complaint prevention.

◆ Service recovery is a tool for complaint management. Use it quickly; use it well.

◆ Leading up is a powerful tool for passing the baton between team members as the patient moves through the system.

REFERENCES

King, M. L., Jr. 1967. "The 3 Dimensions of Life." Sermon delivered at the New Covenant Baptist Church, Chicago, April 9.

Mayer, T., and R. J. Cates. 1999. "Service Excellence in Health Care." *Journal of the American Medical Association* 282 (13): 1281–83.

Mayer, T. A., R. J. Cates, M. J. Mastorovich, and D. L. Royalty. 1998. "Emergency Department Patient Satisfaction: Customer Service Training Improves Patient Satisfaction and Ratings of Physician and Nurse Skill." *Journal of Healthcare Management* 43 (5): 427–40.

Peters, T. J., and R. H. Waterman. 2004. *In Search of Excellence: Lessons from America's Best-Run Companies.* New York: Harper Business.

MORE RESOURCES ON EMPOWERMENT

Frieberg, K., and J. Frieberg. 1997. *Nuts! Southwest Airlines' Crazy Recipe for Business and Personal Success.* New York: Broadway Books.

Gitomer, J. 1998. *Customer Satisfaction Is Worthless, Customer Loyalty Is Priceless: How to Make Customers Love You, Keep Them Coming.* Austin, TX: Bard Press.

Zemke, R., and C. R. Bell. 2000. *Knock Your Socks Off Service Recovery.* New York: AMACOM.

Each of these books is excellent and contains helpful sections on service recovery.

CHAPTER 9

A-Team Tool 2—Dealing with the B-Team

The philosopher in all of us knows that the B-Teams cannot be completely avoided—they are simply a part of life. We happen to believe that a careful and thoughtful approach to working with the B-Teams at your organization can help B-Team patients, staff, and bosses move to the A-Team (or at least *act* like A-Teamers for a few hours at work). This second tool in the A-Team Tool Kit, like all of the other tools, is based on the evidence we have collected in our work over a very long time with literally thousands of people.

DEALING WITH THE DIFFICULT (B-TEAM) PATIENT

Having the ability to deal successfully with difficult patients—some would say "B-Team patients"—is a skill that you and each member of your staff need to possess. While similar to service recovery, dealing with difficult patients is done in real time, preferably at the bedside. As mentioned previously, the most important skill, both here and in service recovery, is listening actively, empathetically, and compassionately. Earlier chapters discuss the topic of listening in much more detail, but here is a brief recap: Say "I'm sorry," and do so in a blameless way.

Learning How to Say You Are Sorry

None of the sentences that follow apportion blame; they simply acknowledge the patient's or family's concerns and indicate you're sorry they feel the way they do.

- "I'm sorry you feel the staff weren't listening to you."
- "I'm sorry you feel the doctor didn't communicate well with your father."
- "I'm sorry you feel we've failed to meet your expectations."

"What Can I Do to Make This Right for You?"

This question may seem like stepping on a land mine, bad advice, or a risk management nightmare. However, if you and your staff have learned the blameless apology technique, more than 90 percent of patients or families who have a complaint and are asked, "What can I do to make this right for you?" are likely to have the same response:

"I just don't want it to happen to anyone else."

When you hear this response, a great reply is, "Thank you for letting us know about this issue. I assure you I will follow up and make changes to keep this from happening again."

The Power of "I" and the Elusiveness of "We" and "They"

Much of the language of healthcare has a vaguely elusive nature about it. Think about how many times you hear questions being answered with these responses:

- "Not to my knowledge."
- "Not that I'm aware of."
- "Not that I know of with the data available at the present time."

Small wonder that patients and families find these answers confusing, if not downright evasive. Similarly, notice how we talk about complaints using "they" most often and "we" less often.

- "The staff tell me they didn't lose your valuables."
- "The lab lost your blood sample. They do that all the time."
- "We can't be expected to meet noncritical needs or expectations. After all, we're a hospital, not a four-star hotel."

This sort of language angers normal people—and infuriates B-Team/difficult patients. Instead, use the first-person singular whenever you can:

- "I'm sorry this happened, but I'll take care of it."
- "I apologize to you and your family. I'll look into it and contact you within 48 hours."
- "I'll make the appropriate changes to see that this doesn't happen again."

Use the Volume Control

Difficult patients and families tend to operate at extraordinarily high volume, since they are angry, frustrated, and seemingly at the end of their rope. Often the problem appears to be that we are "on different channels of the radio." We're on channel 1 and they are on channel 2. We can't make out what each other is saying. What's the natural reaction? Speak louder!

But the louder, more obnoxious, and more unreasonable they are, the softer, more quiet, and more reasonable you should become. Dialing your volume down as theirs goes up helps de-escalate the problem.

Use Proactive Body Language

The importance of body language in transmitting messages dates to ancient times, when opening the hands and arms was a gesture used by our ancestors to show they held no weapons and posed no threat. As we note earlier, Mehrabian's (1981) studies show that comprehension of a verbal message is driven more by visual clues than by the words used. When people are angry with you, they tend to point, gesticulate, and step forward. Rather than match the behavior of angry people, use the power of your body language to a positive, proactive effect: Instead of crossing your arms in a closed, negative posture, open your hands, arms, and facial expression to indicate concern, sympathy, empathy, and openness. Maintaining eye contact, nodding and saying "yes" when they express their concerns, leaning closer at important times, and gesturing with open palms can all be ways to accentuate the positive, even with angry patients.

Remember: You Are Onstage

The Walt Disney Company uses the onstage/offstage analogy to emphasize the performance aspect of service to their "cast members." By not calling them employees, the company reminds staff that they should always remain "in character" when they are "onstage," in front of the public. The problem in healthcare is that you are *always* onstage, except perhaps when you are off-duty in the staff lounge or in the office with the door closed. Most of your staff will encounter angry patients and their families either at the bedside or at the nursing station. Help them understand that these and most other locations in the healthcare setting are onstage in that other patients, families, and fellow healthcare workers are observing these interactions.

Similarly, use the onstage concept to recruit allies by being unfailingly professional, calm, courteous, and compassionate—even in the face of anger and resentment. We have received many letters, voice mails, and e-mails that began, "I want to compliment your staff for being highly professional in a difficult situation I witnessed."

Take the Sail Out of Their Wind

The old adage "Take the wind out of their sails" is unfortunately inaccurate. After all, the complaining patients or families have a seemingly inexhaustible wind supply. Their wind is precisely the problem. Instead, take the *sail* out of their *wind*. In other words, don't give them anything to blow *against*. If there is no resistance to the wind, the ship won't move off course when those ill winds blow.

How do we take the sail out of their wind? Try the following steps:

- *Don't interrupt.* If you ask patients, they'll tell you that healthcare staff are notorious for interrupting patients' responses to the questions they are asked. As we mention in a previous chapter, healthcare professionals tend to interrupt patients within less than a minute of the time they start talking. Let them tell their story, interrupting only at key points to clarify important information.
- *Don't resist.* This is usually not the time to confront them with the facts. When they say they waited 1 hour and 48 minutes for a chest X-ray and you total the time and say it was "only" 1 hour and 37 minutes, it doesn't help. Let them win on the small points so you can concentrate on the big ones.

- *Focus on their concerns.* As patients tell their stories about their journey through healthcare, they almost always provide a certain amount of extraneous detail. Sift through these details to focus on their areas of concern.
- *Focus on expectations.* Ask patients and family members how the hospital failed to meet their expectations. Many patients are seemingly angry about everything, particularly if they feel their dignity has been compromised. Help them focus their expectations. This approach often requires taking the sail out of their wind and then returning their attention to specific expectations.
- *Recognize crusaders.* Some of these folks are so foam-at-the-mouth outraged that they are a tirade in search of an audience. You are the audience. Complainers can become crusaders who seem possessed of an almost evangelical desire to proselytize. (When they have a notebook in which they have catalogued their concerns, you are in particularly troubled waters.)
- *Do your homework.* Whenever possible, review the chart and speak to the healthcare workers involved in the patient's care for their perspective on the encounter. Doing your homework up front saves time in future meetings.
- *Come to closure.* By doing your homework, preparing carefully, and listening empathetically and skillfully, you should be able to resolve complaints at the initial meeting in the majority of cases. Restate the patient/family concerns, express an apology, and state an action plan for follow-up if needed. Send a note of closure, along with a business card, to the patient.

DEALING WITH B-TEAM MEMBERS

One of the questions we are asked most often is, "How do I deal with the B-Team members? How can I get them to move to the A-Team?" As we note at the outset of the book, two fundamental truths must be kept in mind when any change in human behavior is sought:

1. All meaningful and lasting change is intrinsically, not extrinsically, motivated.
2. The number one reason to focus on service excellence is that it makes the job easier.

Trying to get someone to change for *your* reasons—doing it because the boss (or anyone else) says so—is virtually condemned to failure. Why? Because people need to be shown that it is *better for them* to change than to continue in their old habits. There has to be not only a wedge, a driving force to move them away from their old behavior, but also a magnet, a force that pulls them toward a better way of doing things (i.e., makes the job easier). So we need to begin with a clear understanding of this psychological insight and show them both the wedge—the B-Team behavior—and the magnet—the A-Team behavior that makes their job easier. The process looks like this:

Be proactive, not reactive.

Don't wait for the B-Team behavior to rear its ugly head; be positive and proactive in promoting service excellence and the A-Team behaviors. Accentuate and celebrate compliments, showing how A-Team behaviors work and how they are rewarded. Give the magnet of A-Team behaviors meaning.

Solicit Team Input

One question leaders face is, "Is this person's behavior my problem, his problem, or a problem for the entire team?" In a confidential and professional manner, seek the view of key members of the team regarding the B-Team member and his behavior. Hold this information in strict confidence, but use it to ensure that you have an accurate sense of the disruption the B-Team member creates. Never say, "Kim told me about what you did to that patient." Make it about the team and its input, not just individual input. Then use the following steps to eliminate the disruption.

Tie the Effects of the B-Team Behavior to the Team

Many leaders and managers make counseling of B-Team members personal: "I want you to do this" or "I don't want you to do that." It is usually better to tie the negative impact of the B-Team behavior to its impact on the overall team and its vision, mission, and strategies. (Of course, it is always gratifying to say, "Exactly how did your kicking this patient in the groin fit in with the team's customer service initiative?")

Given that the team vision, mission, and strategy are mutually developed and agreed on, relating B-Team actions to those team goals can be helpful and keeps any discussion from becoming personal. It also, if done correctly, encourages the B-Team member to improve his performance to better reflect the team's vision, mission, and strategy. Because it has not been made personal, he will be more motivated to improve.

Reflect, Write It Down, Then Act Quickly

Don't let anger or frustration at what often seems like frequent—or even recalcitrant—B-Team behaviors cause you to react out of that anger or frustration. Instead, reflect on what the B-Team member has done, the impact of that action on the rest of the team, and the context in which it has occurred. Take the time to write it down—what happened, its downstream effects, possible course of action, team input—and then decide what to do.

After you've decided your course of action and before you address the issue, it is usually a good idea to outline what you are going to say to the B-Team member, how you are going to say it, what reaction to expect, and how to respond to those reactions. This step shouldn't take more than 72 hours, and then it's time to act quickly and decisively, following your clear plan of action.

No one likes to be the bearer of bad tidings (well, some people do, but that's another topic altogether), but don't put it off. As soon as you know what needs to be said and how to say it—say it.

Be Specific

Too often, leaders counsel others in language that is, at best, imprecise and, at worst, unclear and passive. Specifically, many healthcare leaders and managers are entirely too vague when it comes to giving corrective feedback to staff. Here's an example of the kind of language that is too often used:

> "Hi, how are you, how's the family? Well, I've been talking to the staff, and you know how much we like things to be fine and better, and we were hoping that you could help us make things better through better actions, because when things go better, people feel better and then it is better. And our journey to better is so important! Well, thanks for coming in today."

What did this manager just say? Most people would say, "Nothing!" If you asked the B-Team member what happened in the meeting, she would probably say, "I think I got a raise."

Don't counsel people that way. Be clear, be concise, and be specific. We like the following format, called the Gordon model, which we learned from our great friend and exemplary healthcare leader Dr. Rob Strauss:

> *When you do* x, *it results in* y; *try* z *instead.*

Think about this for a moment. What is x? Clearly, it is the B-Team behavior about which you should give clear and precise detail. What's y? Well, y is the result, the negative effect of the B-Team behavior, whether it is patients' complaints, families' concerns, disruptions to the other staff, risk management concerns, or poor morale. How about z—what's that? Clearly, z is the A-Team behavior you recommend, a concrete example of how to behave differently and the improved impact that results.

Here's a simple example. One B-Team behavior that drives everyone to distraction is showing up late. No one can stand that, because it is rude, disruptive, and intolerable. And yet we seem to keep tolerating it. Here's how you can put the Gordon model into play:

"When you *show up late* (B-Team behavior), it *makes others feel angry* (the clear consequence of the B-Team behavior); try *doing three fewer tasks before leaving for work* (a practical A-Team behavior to keep people on time).

It is a simple yet highly effective formula that translates the B-Team member's chosen actions to specific negative effects while giving him a practical means to fix the problem. The communication should always be terse, focused, and directly to the point. Don't exchange pleasantries—this is a correction, not a catch-up session. Practice this method, teach it to your leaders and managers, and use it in your counseling sessions. It is the first and most important step toward building a culture of accountability.

A Deeper Dive

We are often asked, "Why do you say 'do three fewer tasks'?" The facts are, if they do one less thing, they are just *less late* than usual. If they do two fewer things, they are *almost on time*, but it takes three fewer things to actually get them to the intended destination at the appointed time. And where would people who show up late *rather* be than at work? You know the answer: "Anywhere!" And that means they haven't answered the "deep joy, deep need" question correctly—they're in the wrong line of work.

Give Them a Mentor

All of you have doctors, nurses, laboratory technicians, radiology technicians, and department directors who are widely respected and admired. Some, perhaps in no formal leadership position, are just great people to have in the organization. Others admire, respect, and look up to them as role models. Use these A-Team members in your organization as mentors to the B-Team members. They can have a profound and dramatic impact on your B-Team members by showing them a better and easier way to do things—that is, the magnet A-Team behaviors and habits that make the job easier.

How do we know who the mentors are? Here's a simple exercise you can do with your staff to help them understand it:

"Close your eyes. Now, imagine that you are a patient on the unit in which you work. You have the most serious and terrifying disease that you could possibly have and still be a patient in that unit. When you open your eyes, you will be looking at the particular doctor, nurse, and essential services staff you most, and most desperately, want to be there for you. Open your eyes. Those are your mentors."

Our view is that coaching and mentoring should be a fundamental and much more widely used part of our leadership skills.

Celebrate Success

When the B-Team members start exhibiting A-Team behaviors, it's time to break out the champagne (figuratively, of course) and celebrate it publicly. This is very powerful stuff and a symbol of hope to others. When the most egregious of the B-Team members start behaving differently, people take serious notice. There is also the Machiavellian aspect that the service excellence change is exponentially accelerated when Nurse Ratched, Dr. Torquemada, and Administrator Scrooge start getting compliments.

Be Prepared for Failure—Fire Right

Some staff members don't get it and will never get it. It doesn't mean they are bad people. However, it does often mean they need to be in a different job (following the "deep joy, deep need" theory) or out of healthcare entirely. As the old saying goes, "Some people you don't get even with, but away from." Don't get us wrong—it's never enjoyable to fire or transfer an employee or a colleague, but sometimes it is necessary.

Whereas some B-Team members just need the remedial course in customer service—they need to go back for additional study, counseling, and homework—others simply do not have the servant's heart that is required to be successful in healthcare. *Fire right* means to fire for the right reasons, based on clearly documented patterns demonstrated by the B-Team member that are harming team morale, and to do so for the good of the patients and the team of caregivers.

Make no mistake—your credibility as a leader is in serious jeopardy if you don't have the courage to deal with the B-Team members. If you don't, the team will say, "There are two sets of rules around here—one set for us, and another for Nurse Ratched and Dr. Cranky." As your kids would say, don't go there.

DEALING WITH B-TEAM BOSSES

Sometimes—not infrequently—the revolution comes from within. What do you do if the troops are fired up for customer service but the department director or assistant administrator is not? Happily, customer service is one of those areas where it is better to ask for forgiveness than for permission. If you have staff who want to cultivate ideas for customer service but also have managers who pose an obstacle, there are ways to cultivate creativity without mutiny.

First, reach down in the organization, not to meddle or micromanage but to show that service excellence is an organizational passion, not a departmental initiative. Leadership team meetings should emphasize this philosophy and stress that you want to hear creative ideas and success stories from throughout the organization.

Second, be aware and tolerant that managers are, of necessity and by nature, at different stages in their learning curves regarding service excellence. Many of them need their own mentors when it comes to nurturing and encouraging A-Team behaviors.

Third, we cannot overemphasize the importance of being visible, vocal, and unceasing in your commitment to service. Making service rounds in the patient care areas and asking patients, "How can we do this better?" to develop as clear an understanding as possible of how the service is delivered is essential to infusing the organization with a commitment to service. Your time is very valuable, but it is never better spent than when seeing and being seen by the patients and the staff who serve them.

Fourth, just as you encourage your staff to be specific with B-Team employees, so should you be with your leadership team. The Gordon model works as well for leaders as it does for employees.

Finally, as we discuss in Chapter 13, it is critical that you *hire right* when you select members of your management team. Ask potential department directors and assistant/associate administrators open-ended yet penetrating questions about their commitment to service excellence, including examples of how they've handled difficult service problems well and references you can contact regarding their commitment to service. They'll get the message—in this organization, service is essential, not optional.

SURVIVAL SKILLS SUMMARY

◆ It is not enough to recognize B-Team members, patients, and bosses; we also must learn how to deal with them in an effective and efficient fashion.
◆ Just as there are B-Team members, there are also B-Team (difficult) patients.
◆ Dealing with the B-Team patient requires taking several steps, including
   1. using a blameless apology to say you are sorry that things have gotten off track;
   2. asking "What can I do to make this right with you?";
   3. using the powerful language of "I" instead of the vague "they";
   4. using the volume control—the louder they get, the more reasonable you get;
   5. remembering that you are onstage and that healthcare customer service is performance art; and
   6. taking the sail out of their wind.
◆ Dealing with B-Team members requires a clear statement of the problematic behavior, which is tied to the team's mission.
◆ Use the Gordon model: When you do x, it results in y; try z instead.
◆ The B-Team behavior is x, the impact on the team is y, and a suggested A-Team behavior to fix the problem is z.
◆ If the Gordon model doesn't work, assign B-Team members a mentor—a trusted A-Team member—to work with and model their behavior after.
◆ If *that* doesn't work, have the courage to act—fire right. Fire for the right reasons, based on clearly documented patterns demonstrated by the B-Team member, and do so for the good of the patients and the team of caregivers.
◆ Managing B-Team bosses who preach service but practice the opposite must also be dealt with.

REFERENCE

Mehrabian, A. 1981. *Silent Messages: Implicit Communication of Emotions and Attitude.* Chicago: Aldine-Atherton.

MORE RESOURCES ON DEALING WITH THE B-TEAM

Mayer, T. 2010. "Dealing with B Team Members." *Healthcare Executive* 25 (5): 52–54.

Mayer, T., J. Kaplan, R. W. Strauss, and R. J. Cates. 2014. "Customer Service in Emergency Medicine." In *Strauss and Mayer's Emergency Department Management*, edited by R. W. Strauss and T. A. Mayer. New York: McGraw-Hill.

CHAPTER 10

A-Team Tool 3—
Patient Satisfaction Coaching

If we blindfolded a pilot, how well do you think he or she would fly the plane? Would you fly an airline that blindfolds its pilots? Of course not. Pick your favorite quarterback—Peyton Manning, his brother Eli, Andrew Luck, Tom Brady, Aaron Rodgers, Robert Griffin III, Colin Kaepernick—they are all great athletes, but put blinders on them and see how well they read their progressions in the passing game with no peripheral vision. Take any activity, sport, or profession that requires a high degree of skill and relies on immediate feedback to judge progress, and then deprive the person of their "sight" or "feel." The results will predictably plummet.

To relate this analogy to healthcare, how many of us are using all of our resources to assess our performance in offering the best customer service for patients? Establishing and maintaining accountability for service requires immediate and actionable feedback from all possible sources to identify and correct any efforts that do not improve service.

Those organizations that don't use the open-book test approach discussed in Chapter 6 are depriving themselves of the opportunity to know how they will be assessed as well as the chance to adequately prepare for the "test." Focused patient satisfaction coaching blends the open-book test approach with a regular, data- and evidence-based method of using our survey scores not only to measure our progress (or lack thereof) but also to develop *specific* A-Team behaviors, scripts, and processes. Focused coaching of healthcare staff is thus based on using the measureable results published regularly along with patient complaints and compliments to guide our activities related to the current situation.

Here are the basic steps of focused patient satisfaction coaching:

1. Start with the open-book test and huddle-up approaches we discuss in Chapter 6.
2. The target score is almost always set for the unit or product line and is usually set on a percentile basis to compare one's organization with other (preferably like) hospitals (e.g., 75th percentile).
3. The percentile score should be converted to a raw score using the scale of the survey (HCAHPS, Press Ganey, Professional Research Consultants [PRC], National Research Corporation–Picker, etc.). This step is necessary so the team knows the specific raw score needed to hit the target percentile.
4. The scores should be broken out by question and trended over time.
5. Rising scores and increased compliments should be analyzed to identify the A-Team behaviors, scripts, and processes that led to them.
6. Falling or stalled scores (and increases in complaints) should be analyzed to discern focused coaching efforts toward making the job easier.
7. In addition to the open-book test approach to the survey questions, all free-text responses to the survey (both positive and negative), as well as compliment and complaint letters, e-mails, phone calls, and other communications, must be included as part of focused patient satisfaction coaching.

Taking all of these steps will have the secondary effect of improving the scores.

Note that a blanket mandate to "Get your scores up!" never works. It refers to an important cause, but it is too vague to be meaningful. On the other hand, adopting a focused coaching strategy for a specific question—for example, to improve scores related to "Doctor was informative regarding care"—usually does work. There must be a specific area of focus that is clear and actionable. (This is also true of any other specific, focused question on any survey.)

The huddle-up approach designs A-Team words and actions around those questions. For example, following are the core areas of behavior that one survey explores to assess the physicians and nurses providing service to patients in the emergency department (ED):

Physicians	Nurses
Courtesy	Courtesy
Took time to listen	Took time to listen
Informative	Informative
Concern for comfort	Attention to needs Concern for privacy

You may ask, "But isn't there also an 'overall' score for each?" Yes, there is, but that overall score is simply the numerical average of the component questions. In the case of physicians, the scores can often be reported for the individual physician who provided the service. These scores can then be used to coach the physician with specific goals toward improvement.

(Nurses' scores are not currently listed in most surveys by individual provider, but the overall scores are provided, as are scores by time of the shift. These scores can be used for focused coaching of nurses and support staff to improve patients' perceptions of their care.)

How do you use percentile scores to frame your focused patient satisfaction coaching course for each clinician? (In the following discussion, taken from the Press Ganey survey, it is important to understand the distinction between *percentile scores,* shown on the left-hand side of exhibits 10.1 and 10.2, which are based on national averages, and *raw scores,* shown in the boxes, which are a numerical average of the scores, typically a Likert scale that ranges from 1 [poor] to 5 [excellent], which are weighted as follows: 1 = 0; 2 = 25; 3 = 50; 4 = 75; 5 = 100.) Here, we compare the scores of Physician 1, Dr. Jones, with those of Physician 2, Dr. Smith, before each has undergone focused patient satisfaction coaching.

Dr. Jones's data are provided in Exhibit 10.1. Look at the top row of scores first. Her target percentile scores have been set at the 85th percentile. To meet the 85th percentile target, Dr. Jones would need to achieve the target raw scores shown in the first-row boxes.

The second row of scores shows Dr. Jones's actual raw scores, including her overall raw score of 86.3. That overall raw score corresponds to a 66th percentile score.

Although Dr. Jones's overall score is at the 66th percentile—well below the target percentile score—she actually has been partially successful at achieving her goal of scoring at the 85th percentile. For example, looking more closely at Dr. Jones's scores, we see that she scored well on the "courtesy" and "took time to listen" measures. Not only did she exceed the 85th percentile in these areas, but she

Exhibit 10.1: Focused Patient Satisfaction Coaching, Physician 1

	Courtesy	Listen	Inform	Comfort	Overall
Target: 85th Percentile	90.1	88.3	86.8	87.2	88.0
Actual: 66th Percentile	90.6	89.1	82.8	82.8	86.3

exceeded the 90th percentile. On these two measures, Dr. Jones is an A-Team physician. However, the scores related to "keeping patients informed" and "showing concern for their comfort" have lowered the overall score dramatically. In future focused patient satisfaction coaching sessions, the leader should focus on those areas for improvement, making sure to compliment this doctor for how high the scores were on the "courtesy" and "took time to listen" measures.

Now let's look at Physician 2, Dr. Smith (see Exhibit 10.2). This physician's overall score is at the 77th percentile, but, in the opposite trend of Dr. Jones's scores, it is "courtesy" and "took time to listen" that are pulling Dr. Smith's overall score down, whereas "kept informed regarding care" and "concern for comfort" are at the highest level. Dr. Smith's efforts in the latter two areas should be celebrated, while the first two areas need improvement, which should be the subject of focused patient satisfaction coaching.

A wise leader can combine the A-Team attributes of Dr. Jones and Dr. Smith. How? Identify what each is doing in his and her areas of strength to help the other. Think about it—if you took the best of the best of these two docs and shared them, instead of having one 66th percentile doc and one 77th percentile doc, you would have two docs scoring well above the 90th percentile. This is the concept behind focused patient satisfaction coaching (Mayer et al. 2014). Instead of simply looking at the overall score, break down the component questions and analyze what is working well (scores above the target raw and percentile scores) and celebrate those A-Team behaviors with both the individual doctor and the entire team. Conversely, take the relevant questions where the clinician falls below the target and provide her with focused coaching to improve, including assigning her a mentor whose behaviors and language are producing excellent results.

The same method can be applied to efforts to improve the perception of service in other patient satisfaction surveys. For example, for PRC scores, three "key drivers" are identified on a statistical basis, which for each ED are the main determinants of the overall score. By focusing on these key drivers and coaching the staff to

Exhibit 10.2: Focused Patient Satisfaction Coaching, Physician 2

	Courtesy	Listen	Inform	Comfort	Overall
Target: 85th Percentile ➡	90.1	88.3	86.8	87.2	88.0
Actual: 77th Percentile ➡	88.5	86.5	88.0	87.0	87.0

address them—simply another form of focused patient satisfaction coaching—the scores can be improved. Exhibit 10.3 shows an example from BestPractices of using the key driver "respect for patient privacy" to focus our staff coaching and the dramatic results that can occur.

As we discuss in more detail in Chapter 15, "Flow and the Psychology of Waiting," focusing efforts on length of stay and flow parameters can also be a very effective way to improve satisfaction (Exhibit 10.4).

THE ROLE OF DATA MINING IN FOCUSED PATIENT SATISFACTION COACHING

Ask yourself these questions: Do you manage by data or by anecdote? (And no, the plural of "anecdote" is not "data.") Do you primarily use objective or subjective units of measure? Do you hold your leaders and managers accountable? How often? What tools are they given when progress toward specified metrics is stalled?

Exhibit 10.3: Key Drivers of Excellence for IFH, by Month

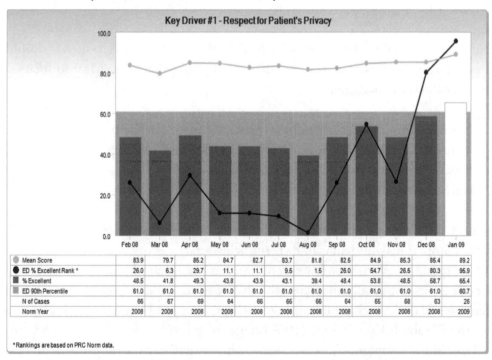

	Feb 08	Mar 08	Apr 08	May 08	Jun 08	Jul 08	Aug 08	Sep 08	Oct 08	Nov 08	Dec 08	Jan 09
⬤ Mean Score	83.9	79.7	85.2	84.7	82.7	83.7	81.8	82.5	84.9	85.3	85.4	89.2
⬤ ED % Excellent Rank *	26.0	6.3	29.7	11.1	11.1	9.5	1.5	26.0	54.7	26.5	80.3	95.9
■ % Excellent	48.5	41.8	49.3	43.8	43.9	43.1	39.4	48.4	53.8	48.5	58.7	65.4
▦ ED 90th Percentile	61.0	61.0	61.0	61.0	61.0	61.0	61.0	61.0	61.0	61.0	61.0	60.7
N of Cases	66	67	69	64	66	65	66	64	65	68	63	26
Norm Year	2008	2008	2008	2008	2008	2008	2008	2008	2008	2008	2008	2009

*Rankings are based on PRC Norm data.

Source: Professional Research Corporation report for Inova Fairfax Hospital. Used with permission.

Exhibit 10.4: Improving PRC Survey Scores

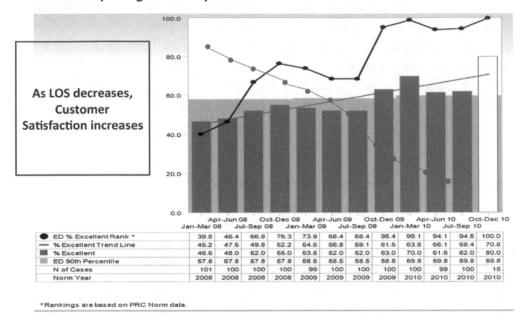

	Jan-Mar 08	Apr-Jun 08	Jul-Sep 08	Oct-Dec 08	Jan-Mar 09	Apr-Jun 09	Jul-Sep 09	Oct-Dec 09	Jan-Mar 10	Apr-Jun 10	Jul-Sep 10	Oct-Dec 10
● ED % Excellent Rank *	39.8	46.4	66.8	76.3	73.9	68.4	68.4	95.4	99.1	94.1	94.5	100.0
— % Excellent Trend Line	45.2	47.5	49.8	52.2	54.5	56.8	59.1	61.5	63.8	66.1	68.4	70.8
■ % Excellent	46.5	48.0	52.0	55.0	53.5	52.0	52.0	63.0	70.0	61.6	62.0	80.0
▨ ED 90th Percentile	57.8	57.8	57.8	57.8	58.5	58.5	58.5	58.5	59.8	59.8	59.8	59.8
N of Cases	101	100	100	100	99	100	100	100	100	99	100	15
Norm Year	2008	2008	2008	2008	2009	2009	2009	2009	2010	2010	2010	2010

*Rankings are based on PRC Norm data.

Source: Professional Research Corporation report for Inova Fairfax Hospital. Used with permission.

In addition to all of the survey-specific data that are provided to us, we should also take into account three areas ripe for data mining that are critical to focused patient satisfaction coaching:

1. Free-text comments, a part of most surveys, in which the patient or family writes specific feedback to the questions asked in the survey
2. Patient compliments (all sources: e-mail, voice mail, letter, etc.)
3. Patient complaints (all sources)

Specifically, the compliments will identify A-Team behaviors being demonstrated, and the complaints will delineate B-Team behaviors.

Our experience, with very few exceptions, has been that physicians, nurses, and other caregivers universally appreciate the chance to see the data provided in focused patient satisfaction coaching to improve their practice. To be sure, there is always a bit of the Elisabeth Kübler-Ross (1969) stages of grieving (denial, anger, bargaining, depression, acceptance/peace) evident when negative data are presented. That said, the soonest and most clearly we as leaders can convey what the data show, the more quickly we can help the members of our team move to more solid footing when it comes to the details of making their jobs easier through the disciplines of service excellence.

Most of us would say we have a fierce, metrics-driven focus on delivering the results that matter. If that's true, why aren't we systematically providing our staff with evidence-based tools and techniques for focused patient satisfaction coaching? You're likely to see that employee satisfaction rises when you put the right armamentarium into the hands of the folks in the trenches of patient care. For example, after we introduced focused patient satisfaction coaching to one experienced physician, his scores soared, and the satisfaction of the nurses who worked with him did as well. He came to us and said, "Bob and Thom, for 20 years, people have been yelling at me to 'get your scores up!' But you guys showed me *how* to get my scores up." It was very gratifying for us to hear—and it will be for you as well.

SURVIVAL SKILLS SUMMARY

♦ Establishing and maintaining accountability for service requires immediate and actionable feedback to identify and correct any efforts that do not improve service.
♦ The basic steps of focused patient satisfaction coaching are as follows:
  1. Start with the open-book test and huddle-up approaches discussed in Chapter 6.
  2. The target score is almost always set for the unit or product line and is usually set on a percentile basis to compare one's organization with other (preferably like) hospitals (e.g., 75th percentile).
  3. The percentile score should be converted to a raw score using the scale of the survey (HCAHPS, Press Ganey, Professional Research Consultants, National Research Corporation–Picker, etc.).
  4. The scores should be broken out by question and trended over time.
  5. Rising scores and increased compliments should be analyzed to identify the A-Team behaviors, scripts, and processes that led to them.
  6. Falling or stalled scores (and increases in complaints) should be analyzed to discern focused coaching efforts toward making the job easier.
Taking all of these steps will have the secondary effect of improving the scores. Note that a blanket mandate to "Get your scores up!" never works. It states an important cause, but it is too vague to be meaningful. On the other hand, adopting a focused coaching strategy for a specific question, for example to improve scores related to "Doctor was informative regarding care," usually

does work. There must be a specific area of focus that is clear and actionable. (This is also true of any other specific, focused question on any survey.)

◆ In addition to the open-book test approach to the survey questions, all free-text responses to the survey (both positive and negative) as well as compliment and complaint letters, e-mails, phone calls, and other communications—the results of data mining—must also be included in focused patient satisfaction coaching.

REFERENCES

Kübler-Ross, E. 1969. *On Death and Dying.* New York: Simon and Schuster.

Mayer, T., J. Kaplan, R. W. Strauss, and R. J. Cates. 2014. "Customer Service in Emergency Medicine." In *Strauss and Mayer's Emergency Department Management,* edited by R. W. Strauss and T. A. Mayer. New York: McGraw-Hill.

CHAPTER 11

A-Team Tool 4—Rounding

One of the most powerful tools available to leaders and managers is rounding. *Rounding* is an evidence-based and disciplined process by which information is shared through two-way communication between leaders and managers and the patients, families, team members, and physicians they serve.

Rounding puts us in touch with our two most critical customers: those who are internal and those who are external. The external customers are, of course, our patients and their families, and they serve as the *voice of the customer* (VOC). But it is important to recall that rounding also puts us in touch with the internal customers—the team we work with on a daily basis, including our staff and our physicians, to meet and exceed the expectations of our patients.

The importance of the leader being visible to "the troops" is as ancient as warfare. There are countless examples and quotes from field commanders attesting to the value of those who are charged with making difficult leadership decisions being close to those who will enact those decisions. World War II Generals George S. Patton Jr., Terry de la Mesa Allen, Brute Krulak, and Theodore Roosevelt Jr. were perhaps the best examples of those who "led from the front" by constantly putting themselves in a position to hear the thoughts and concerns of their frontline troops. To extend the analogy, few commanders who "hole up" at command posts or headquarters distant from the action have ever been successful—whether in business, battle, or healthcare.

To be sure, there is a discrete, if hidden, cost to spending excessive time in the office or in meetings. Failing to keep in contact with those we serve puts us at serious risk of isolation—not a healthy strategy in the perpetual whitewater of change in which we now find ourselves. More than 30 years ago, Peters and Waterman (2007) advised leaders of the wisdom of MBWA, or Management by Wandering Around. But even then, MBWA was never intended as a casual stroll through the premises, but rather a disciplined approach to stay in close contact with the core business.

TYPES OF ROUNDING

We have identified three types of rounding:

◆ *Rounding on yours.* Leaders round on their own units to hear feedback from patients, the team, and the physicians.
◆ *Rounding on next.* Leaders, physicians, and nurses round on patients admitted to the inpatient units or transferred to the next level of care (including, paradoxically, those who have been discharged).
◆ *Rounding transitions.* Physicians, nurses, and other clinical team members conduct sign-out rounds (bedside rounds to transfer care from one provider or group of providers to another) and bedside shift-change reports.

Rounding on Yours

Leader rounding is a core concept of the Studer Group's Evidence-Based Leadership program. Rounding on yours requires leaders to round on patients, staff, and physicians on their unit on a regular basis and to systematically record the results of rounding to improve both service and operations over time. The disciplined use of rounding has shown consistent and dramatic results, including improvements in service scores, length of stay, number of people who left without treatment, and employee and physician satisfaction (Baker 2012). Rounding on units to speak to the staff is best done on an unannounced or random basis, if the leader wants the clearest view of what is actually occurring on the units.

However, some advocate that while rounding should be a part of the leader's regular schedule, it should occur in a more formal, planned fashion. While the latter perhaps gives a less candid view of operations, some unit leaders prefer it so they can showcase the proud and positive accomplishments the team has made. Our view is that rounding on yours should be a part of the daily fabric of the schedule, and announcing ahead of time that it will occur can have the feel of formality—and rarity—that often defeats the primary purpose of the discipline, which is to keep leaders close to the action and close to the patients, staff, and physicians.

Healthcare systems that have embraced rounding build it into every leader's and manager's daily schedule. They do so, for example, by having leaders ask specific questions requiring that rounding logs be kept and reviewed by senior leaders to keep them in touch with the process.

Rounding on Your Teams

Some typical rounding questions for leaders to ask their unit teams include the following:

- What's going well today?
- What needs improvement?
- Are there team members I need to compliment?
- What do you want to see more of?
- What do you want to see less of?

Rounding on Your Patients

The Studer Group (2014) offers a number of tips for rounding on patients:

- Round on staff prior to rounding on patients. Connect the dots on the areas of focus for rounding on patients. Staff should view rounding on patients as a positive activity because of the feedback the leader shares with them from their patients.
- Know the patient (name, diagnosis, physician, nature of visit, etc.).
- Limit the areas of focus for follow-up rounding (address key driver of patient satisfaction, validate staff's use of key behaviors, etc.) to no more than two.
- Sit down to let the patient know you are listening.
- Set the expectation of time to be spent with the patient up front.
- Provide the patient with specific information when leading up the staff. For example, "Today, Jen will be taking care of you. She is an excellent nurse, and I have worked with her for ten years. I would want her to be my nurse if I were having this procedure."
- Instead of using direct, staccato questions ("Do you know who your nurse is?" "What procedure are you having?" "Have things been explained to you?"), engage the patient and family in a conversation, and work these questions in naturally.
- Dig deeper into specific issues—use phrases such as "Please tell me more about that" or "I am pleased to hear you think your nurse is great. What is she doing to make you feel that way?"
- Use closing statements. When a leader asks a patient, "Is there anything I can do for you before I leave?" it tells the patient that the leader cares and the patient's input is important.

- Communicate outcomes with staff following any interaction with patients.
- Information that is documented should include a patient identifier, feedback on areas of focus, staff and physicians to recognize, and items for follow-up.

This list helps address the "how" of rounding on patients, but it is also important to have parameters on "how many" patients should be visited on rounds. Studer (2003) recommends the parameters shown in Exhibit 11.1 (which vary by unit or practice).

As rounding becomes a part of the culture and fabric of the organization, charge nurses should round hourly with the staff to keep abreast of the situation on the unit. This practice can be very helpful on units where the demand–capacity balance is fluid, such as an emergency department (ED), operating suite, or intensive care unit (ICU), or where situational awareness is critical.

Exhibit 11.1: Parameters for Rounding on Patients

Patient Type	Evidence-Based Practice Parameters
Inpatient	Initially, at least once during hospitalization, priority is the following: • Upon admission • Follow-up • Prior to discharge • Patients being held in the ED greater than *x* hours for admission Goal is 100% of patients each day
Critical Care	100% of patients and/or families each day 100% of patients prior to transfer from unit
Emergency Department	25% of treat-and-release patients 100% of patients holding for an inpatient bed Waiting room: • Every 30 minutes if arrival-to-DC time is <150 minutes • Every hour if arrival-to-DC time is >150 minutes
Outpatients	25% of patients daily 100% of new patients to episodic care (rehab, infusion, etc.)
Medical Practice	100% of new patients 100% of patients in waiting room more than 30 minutes

Rounding on Your Physicians

Without question, one of the distinguishing features of "great," as opposed to "good," healthcare organizations is their ability to effectively engage physicians in the evidence-based change efforts. Engagement requires involving them at every stage of the process, and that requires creating regular conversations with them, just as we do with our patients and our team. The engagement effort starts with orientation of new physicians, as it establishes cultural expectations at the outset of their relationship with the hospital, healthcare system, or medical group.

Who should present to physician orientation regarding the culture of engagement? Ideally, all members of the C-suite should take at least a few minutes to deliver the following messages:

- You are the most important resource we have.
- Your care of our patients is paramount, both clinically and from a service standpoint.
- Our culture is evidence based and disciplined in nature and is tied to our mission, vision, and values.
- You will be expected to support our mission, vision, and values, in return for which we will do everything in our power to support you in these efforts.
- We believe regular communication with you is essential to our joint success in meeting and exceeding our patients' expectations.
- Meeting and exceeding those expectations can only occur when we operate under an open-door policy when it comes to communication. If you have a problem, let us know about it in real time.
- We will be rounding on you and your colleagues to ensure that there is a foundation of regular communication and trust on which to build our relationship with you.

Rounding can occur in many ways, but it starts with rounding on the units themselves, where physicians are often rounding on their patients. If a leader has responsibility for the operating suite, rounding in the surgeons' lounge is an excellent way to gauge what issues and concerns they have. In addition, rounding by attending department and section meetings on a regular basis is a good way to stay in touch with the needs of those physicians. Meeting regularly with the medical directors or chairs of various departments and sections paves a two-way street for communication with medical staff leadership. (While the board's medical executive committee also provides an opportunity for communication, highly successful leaders have already prepared key medical staff leaders who will make or influence important decisions by "teeing up" those issues carefully to achieve the best outcomes for the patients, physicians, and healthcare system.)

We should also not neglect a time-honored, but unfortunately increasingly rare, opportunity to round on physicians, which is to make sure that medical staff have a place to eat meals in the hospital cafeteria, whether in a separate medical staff area or a small area within the main cafeteria. And in those areas, leaders should make sure to eat meals there with the physicians to hear their candid concerns and perspectives on how best to improve hospital operations and service.

The effect of rounding on medical staff satisfaction and loyalty is dramatic. Exhibit 11.2 shows that the results of frequent rounding on physicians are positive and predictable.

Rounding on Next

Whereas rounding on yours means ensuring that you hear the perspective of patients and families while they are on your unit or units for which you are responsible, rounding on next refers to taking a regular and disciplined approach to "catching up" with those same patients and families after they have moved to the next area of their care. We first learned of the importance of rounding on next

---

Exhibit 11.2: Rounding for Outcomes: Leaders Rounding on Staff and Physicians

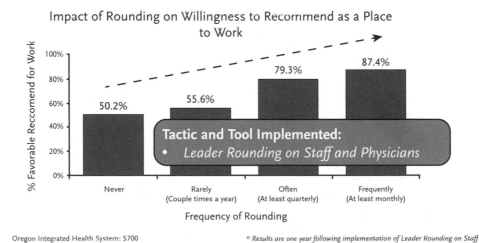

Oregon Integrated Health System: 5700 employees

* Results are one year following implementation of Leader Rounding on Staff and Physicians. Staff and physicians rounded on at least monthly had the highest satisfactin levels.

Source: Studer Group. Used with permission.

---

when we began rounding on a small group of patients admitted from the ED to the inpatient units. We found catching up with them to be an extremely powerful activity by which to initiate change, both for the patients and for the physicians and nurses who care for the patients.

The principle is simple: Leaders, doctors, and nurses keep a log of the patients admitted for whom they have personally cared and who have since been admitted to the hospital (in the case of the ED) or transferred to the next level of care (for inpatients). Once a week, physicians and nurses are encouraged to round on these patients—simply revisit them, check on their progress, and determine how they might have improved their care or better exceeded the patient's expectations.

For example, ICU nurses and physicians should visit patients who have been transferred to step-down units or monitored beds. Operating room nurses should visit patients they cared for on the surgical floor. This practice helps establish a continuity of care that is extraordinarily helpful, both to the patients and to the providers.

But the most sustaining benefit of rounding on next is the genuine respect and gratitude these patients show, almost without exception, when the staff visit them. Indeed, in some cases, such patients become gracious friends. By far the most common reaction we get from patients when we round on next is, "I can't believe you took the time to check on me. And I am so glad you did, because I was so sick down in the ED, I didn't have a chance to tell you how much I appreciated all you did for me." And we also get to hear the "six most important words" an emergency physician ever gets to hear: "Do you have a private practice?" Because when you hear that, patients are telling you that you are their vision of what a *real doctor* should be.

We believe that rounding on next is one of the most powerful but underused tools in the A-Team Tool Kit. We require it of all of our physicians, nurse practitioners, and physician assistants. Not only does it provide tremendous gratification for our clinicians and create loyalty among our patients, but it also is yet another way we can systematically hear the feedback of the patients and their families.

Rounding on next also includes postdischarge or postprocedure phone calls, since these are simply additional ways we can create an ongoing relationship with the customer and hear feedback on the care that was provided.

Rounding Transitions

As we discuss earlier in the book and in more detail in Chapter 15, on hardwiring flow, healthcare is a series of service transitions from one provider or area of care to another. The smooth management of those transitions is essential for the patients, the families, and the service providers themselves. Sign-out rounds and bedside shift-change reports are additional tools that help ensure that we are effectively "passing the baton" to our team members. As a part of their orientation and onboarding to BestPractices, we make sure our physicians are aware that it is our expectation that at change of shift, they go to each patient room and introduce to the patient the clinician who will be replacing them. For example:

> "Mrs. Ramirez, this is Dr. Lo, and he is the emergency physician who will be responsible for completing your care, since I am going off duty now. I have briefed him fully on your care, but I wanted to make sure you had a chance to meet him. He is one of our best doctors, and he will take great care of you."

As with rounding on next, this powerful tool has been neglected in far too many hospitals. It should not be, however. Not only does it give the patient a chance to meet the emergency physician coming on duty, but it also gives us the chance to lead that clinician up in a meaningful way. In addition, it gives us the chance to discuss the pertinent clinical and nonclinical aspects of the patients' care. This is an essential service transition and one that dramatically improves both patient and staff satisfaction. Further, it ensures a clear and consistent understanding among the caregivers and patients of what is to happen.

Bedside change-of-shift reports by the nursing staff are also an excellent example of rounding transitions and should be used on every unit in the hospital. These reports by the nursing staff ensure not only that those staff members share all pertinent information for an evidence-based handoff but also that the patient (and family, if present) is aware of the effective information transfer and has a chance to update and/or correct any of that information.

SURVIVAL SKILLS SUMMARY

- ◆ Rounding is one of the most powerful tools in healthcare because it systematically keeps leaders in touch with the voice of the customer, including patients, families, team members, and physicians.
- ◆ Rounding is an evidence-based and disciplined process by which information is shared through two-way communication between leaders and managers and the patients, families, team members, and physicians they serve.
- ◆ There are three types of rounding: rounding on yours, rounding on next, and rounding transitions.

- Rounding on yours is a disciplined way of staying in touch with the units or areas for which we are responsible and includes rounding on team members, patients, and physicians.
- The results of rounding on yours should be captured on rounding logs and analyzed for trends, advances, and results.
- Rounding on next ensures that we and the staff we lead either visit or telephone the patients after their care has been transitioned to the next level.
- Rounding on next not only creates patient loyalty but also increases staff satisfaction and is one of the most valuable yet underused tools we have available.
- Rounding transitions includes both sign-out rounds for physicians and bedside shift-change reports for the nursing staff.

REFERENCES

Baker, S. J. 2012. "Hourly Rounding in the Emergency Department: How to Accelerate Results." *Journal of Emergency Nursing* 38 (1): 69–72.

Peters, T., and R. H. Waterman. 2007. *In Search of Excellence: Lessons from America's Best-Run Companies.* New York: Collins Business Essentials.

Studer, Q. 2014. *A Culture of High Performance: Achieving Higher Quality at a Lower Cost.* Gulf Breeze, FL: Fire Starter Press.

———. 2003. *Hardwiring Excellence.* Gulf Breeze, FL: Fire Starter Press.

MORE RESOURCES ON ROUNDING

Ambrose, S. E. 2003. *Citizen Soldiers: The US Army from the Normandy Beaches to the Bulge to the Surrender of Germany.* New York: Simon and Schuster.

Astor, G. 2000. *Terrible Terry Allen: Combat General of WWII—the Life of an American Soldier.* New York: Ballantine.

D'Este, C. 1995. *Patton: A Genius for War.* New York: HarperCollins.

Mayer, T., and K. Jensen. 2009. *Hardwiring Flow: Systems and Processes for Seamless Patient Care.* Gulf Breeze, FL: Fire Starter Press.

CHAPTER 12

A-Team Tool 5—Scripts: Using Language to Improve the Patient Experience

We believe that all language has meaning. But sometimes the language we use (or the way we use it) is interpreted differently than we meant it—an example of the "law of unintended consequences" (Merton 1936). How can we ensure that our language and the meaning taken from it are predictable, reliable, and ultimately in service of both patient care and the ease with which we deliver that care?

WHY SCRIPTS?

We know that the patient's journey through our hospitals and healthcare systems is a series of highly predictable service transitions from people and processes to other people and processes. If we understand those transitions, we can bring a high degree of predictability to the interactions that patients, their families, and our staff have. A concept we call *scripts* or *scripting* helps us recognize this predictability and seeks to design words or phrases that best serve our ability to provide an excellent patient experience.

Dealing with Resistance to Scripts

On the one hand, we ask our staff to accept empowerment, and on the other hand, we give them scripts to follow (albeit those that are meant to provide evidence-based guidelines on how to make our jobs easier). As we've noted, the rulebooks are thin, but there *are* rulebooks. Staff's resistance to being told what things to do and how to do them, even if those actions reliably and predictably make our jobs easier, is understandable. The key is to embrace this paradox and put it to use for us and for our patients.

Consider this statement:

> "First you tell us we are empowered to do whatever is best for the patient, then you try to control what we say and how we say it."

When you hear that, or some variation of it (and you will), here's some language that we have found to be helpful in effectively countering such resistance:

> "Would you take care of a patient in cardiac arrest and not follow the ACLS protocols? Would you care for a trauma patient and not use ATLS guidelines? Would you treat a critically ill or injured child and not use APLS and PALS wisdom? Of course not! Scripts are merely the patient satisfaction equivalents of ACLS, ATLS, and APLS/PALS. It's that simple—and it's that critical."

Especially in situations when resistance is encountered, it is not just acceptable but essential to allow the staff members to adapt, modify, and improve on scripts. They need to be able to put their own touches on scripts from their A-Team language skills. For example, Meryl Streep, George Clooney, and all great actors have scripts they are expected to follow, but all of them make that script "their own" in the way they interpret and deliver their lines. The same is true for healthcare providers, since they are, as we've said before, fundamentally performance artists in the way they deliver the message of compassion and concern. However, not using scripts is not an acceptable solution for the vast majority of healthcare environments.

Investing Time Wisely: "Take 5 for a 5"

When faced with resistance to script creation, using the "take 5 for a 5" approach is one way to help counter that resistance. "Take 5 for a 5" means that it only takes 5 seconds to use an effective script that creates satisfaction levels leading the patient to rank our care as "excellent"—or a 5 on a patient satisfaction scale.

Virtually all healthcare patient satisfaction surveys are based on Likert scales (named for sociologist Rensis Likert, who developed the concept of using numerical scales to rank ordinal data). Most scales range from 1 to 5, with 5 being excellent. It is from this that common expressions such as "drive to a 5" originate.

(The HCAHPS survey asks patients to rate their experience in terms of "Always," "Usually," "Sometimes," or "Never," but the fundamental concept is the same. We suppose you could say "take 4 for a 4" on those scales, but you get the point.)

And yet, despite the ease of creating scripts for better patient satisfaction scores, you no doubt will hear something like this from B-Team members:

"I don't have *time* for this nonsense. Don't you know how *busy* we are?"

Time is among our most precious resources. But B-Team members will twist this logic by saying scripts are a waste of that resource. Is that true? No. The intelligent and effective use of language is actually an *investment* of time, not a waste of time. Communication with our patients and their families is one of the most important things we do. Scripts merely help us most effectively use the time it takes to communicate. How much time does it take to verbalize most scripts? As Exhibit 12.1 shows, good scripts rarely take more than 5 seconds to deliver. (The one exception is discussed below.) So, wisely investing time starts with "take 5 seconds. . . ."

What better investment can we make in healthcare than taking 5 seconds to create satisfied, loyal patients who tell their friends and neighbors, "Wow! They are really nailing it at Memorial Medical Center!" *That* is maximizing ROI.

The exception we mention earlier is when we are delivering difficult or bad news. When that occurs, it is time to sit down, establish physical contact, and take whatever time is necessary to both deliver the news and have time to let the patient and family absorb, react, and ask questions. In these cases, it may take 5 *minutes* or even 50 minutes, but it is also an important investment of our time for the good of the patient.

Exhibit 12.1: Take 5 for a 5

"I don't have *time* for customer service."

It only takes 5 seconds, in most cases, to exceed expectations.	"I am sorry this happened to you, but I am glad I am here to take care of you."
You don't have time *not* to take the time.	"How is your pain after that medication?"
Don't let life be a surprise to you.	"Did that blanket help warm you up, or do you need another?"
Service excellence is a discipline, not a character trait.	"Great news—the tests are negative!"

NOT JUST ANY SCRIPTS . . .

There is a systematic approach to using scripts that includes applying proven methods of communicating that improve the patient experience—evidence-based language (EBL)—and linking the words and phrases we use to those that appear in customer satisfaction surveys—survey-based language (SBL).

Evidence-Based Language in Scripts

Just as evidence-based guidelines and protocols are widely used in clinical settings, scripts allow clinicians to benefit from decades of service experience with patients to guide their language skills. Scripting relies on verbal skills that, through extensive experience, have reliably and predictably managed the service transitions and interactions in a positive fashion by prospectively managing patients' and families' perceptions of care.

EBL serves the following functions in scripts:

1. The focus is on what works.
2. What works is translated into scripts.
3. EBL develops A-Team behaviors into scripts.

Survey-Based Language in Scripts

All healthcare customer service surveys cover the same general areas, including the following:

- Staff cared about you as a person
- Kept informed about delays
- Medical care worth the money charged
- Reasonable length of stay
- Physician and nurses informative about treatments
- Adequacy of information provided to family/friends
- Physician and nurses' attention shown to you
- Courtesy shown to family/friends
- Nurses took problem seriously
- Courtesy of nurses
- Nurses' concern for privacy
- Physician and nurses addressed pain effectively

Whichever survey is administered at your hospital or healthcare system, it should be treated as an open-book test, as we discuss—persuasively, we hope—earlier in the book. All staff members should know the questions that are asked on the survey.

A Deeper Dive

As we have noted previously, the majority of medical schools do not "screen for the customer service gene" in selecting potential medical students. Fortunately, a new trend is taking hold. The Association of American Medical Colleges has instituted the Medical College Admissions Test (MCAT) 2015 Project, which has added an entire section on social and behavioral aspects of care to the benchmark test by which prospective medical students are assessed. Beginning in 2016 and culminating with the graduation class of 2020, all medical students will be evaluated by and educated in a system in which communication skills are more highly valued than in the traditional medical training format. This project has taken an important step toward ensuring that those who will need to communicate the most important information in the most difficult of circumstances have at least the baseline proclivity to practice or interest in practicing effective communication and, perhaps, the skills to do so.

Not only should staff know the questions, but they should also be practicing behaviors and using language reflected in those questions. This is where scripts come in. Scripts are the means by which your staff can "ace the test" because they are made up of SBL that ties the questions on the survey to the specific language used by the staff. The scripts should be designed around the particular questions in the survey to effectively address each area of customer satisfaction. Make the survey work for you, instead of you feeling like you are working for the survey.

SBL serves the following functions in scripts:

1. The focus is on what is being measured.
2. What's measured is then tied to language.
3. SBL anchors A-Team scripts to the details of the survey's language.

Let's say the survey asks, "Did the nurses and doctors keep you informed?" An example of SBL that matches up to the question is, "It is very important to me that we *keep you informed* about your care." Similarly, if the survey asks, "Did the staff take time to answer your questions?" an example of an SBL tie-in is, "Do you have any *questions*? I have plenty of *time*."

As we mention earlier in the book, some surveys (e.g., PRC) rank the questions in terms of key drivers, which statistically rank the questions most likely to drive overall satisfaction. In those cases, particular attention should be given to the key drivers following each reassessment to ensure that the scripts are appropriate to the key drivers. For example, if one of the key drivers is "Concern for privacy," then a script that emphasizes, "Shall I close this door to *ensure your privacy?*" would be appropriate.

Combining EBL and SBL

Combining the EBL and SBL approaches is the most reliable and intelligent method for using this extremely effective tool.[1]

The chart that follows summarizes EBL and SBL functions when combined into scripts:

EBL	SBL
1. Focus is on what works.	Focus is on what is being measured.
2. What works is translated into scripts.	What's measured is then tied to language.
3. Develops A-Team behaviors into scripts.	Anchors A-Team scripts to the details of the survey's language.

In terms of this combination, SBL is an essential tool for matching what works with what's being measured.

DEVELOPING SCRIPTS

While scripts have EBL and SBL as their foundation, they also should be framed by two overarching sets of guidelines: general characteristics of well-formatted scripts and key components for any scripted message.

General Characteristics of Effective Scripts

A well-formulated scripted response is designed to simultaneously accomplish several goals. All scripts should

- be easy and "natural" to use,
- provide consistent approaches to sometimes difficult situations,
- use words that appear in subsequent patient satisfaction surveys,
- communicate what patients want to hear (empathy, concern) in words that are comfortable to use,
- use personal feedback and input from ED team members to hone or improve the scripts, and
- be developed with EBL and SBL approaches, but with *team input.*

Components of Well-Formulated Scripts

Effective scripts are designed to contain most or all of the components shown here (see also Exhibit 12.2 and the "Script Examples" section of the chapter for examples by component):

Component	Words/Phrases
1. Personalizing the provider	*I, we*
2. Personalizing the patient	*You, your*
3. Significance	*It is important because we care about your _____ .*
4. Issue addressed	e.g., *information, privacy, comfort*

Effective communicators share what is important to them. First, providers who use "I" statements or use the words *to me* or *by me* create a personal connection and take personal responsibility for the intention described. Second, when personalizing the action by including *you* or *your,* the patient knows that the actions taken and efforts made by the provider are about the patient, her comfort, her privacy, or another issue the patient is dealing with.

Third, using the words *important to me* or *care about your* lets the other person (patient/family member) know that the issue has significance to the speaker (provider). The fourth component of effective scripts, addressing the issue, offers much more than a routine gesture. For example, simply stating, "I'm closing your curtain" describes the action, but not the intent. Adding the words *for your* **privacy** lets patients know why the action is taken and allows them to recognize the specific way the provider is meeting their needs. Then, when those patients take a survey and are asked about privacy, it is likely that they will answer positively. Phrases such as *I care about your comfort/safety/privacy* or *Your comfort/safety/privacy is important to me*

Exhibit 12.2: Matching Patient Satisfaction Principles to Specific Scripts

Patient Satisfaction Principle	Reason	Script
Privacy	Doors and curtains are closed for privacy, but patients are usually unaware of this intent.	"I am closing your curtain because **I care about your privacy**." Or asking permission, "Would **you** like **me** to close the door for your **privacy**?"
Comfort	Comfort measures are provided without patients' awareness.	"**Your comfort** is **important** to **me**. May **I** get **you** a blanket?"
Anxiety	ED patients are often anxious, in pain, and uncertain about what will transpire.	"I'm sorry you're having <symptoms>. We take care of this all the time and will take excellent care of you."
Informing about treatment delays (3 parts)	Patients and families wait without understanding the reason. Sharing the reason and demonstrating concern dramatically improve patients' perceptions of the providers' level of caring.	Initial interaction, after exam and explanation of next steps: "It is **important** to **me** that **you** are kept **informed**. Do you have any questions?" After updating patient (family) during visit: "Keeping **you informed** is **important** to **me**. Do you have any questions?" At close, after explaining the diagnosis and providing discharge instructions: "As I've mentioned, it is **important** to **me** that **you** have been kept **informed**. Have you been?"
Pain	While eliminating pain is not always possible or appropriate, addressing it always is.	"It is **important** to **me** that **your pain** is addressed. Let's discuss the most appropriate way."
Chronic pain	A few patients have chronic pain syndromes that are difficult to fully address in the ED.	"I'm sorry that you have this pain. While providing your care, I will communicate with your doctor to ensure that your treatment is consistent with your pain management program."

Waits/excellent care	Patients mind waiting less if the providers are courteous and show concern about the wait and the patients believe the wait was worthwhile, that is, the promise of excellent care.	"Hello, I'm <Name>. I'm the physician (nurse, technician, phlebotomist, nurse practitioner, etc.) who will be taking care of you. I'm sorry that you've had to wait. **I intend** to give **you excellent care**."
Courtesy	Patients and their families expect courtesy and concern.	See "AIDET" in Chapter 4: "**Your comfort** is **important** to **me**. May I get you a warm blanket?"
Time taken to listen and address needs	Throughout the interaction, it is critical to patients that their needs are addressed.	Initially: Concisely repeat the patient's complaint and then say, "Have I heard you correctly?" During care or at end: "It is **important** to **me** that **I address your needs** and **answer your questions**. Have I?" "For your safety, let me check your armband and your chart to make sure everything is accurate."
Safety	Avoid sentinel events by ensuring right patient, right procedure.	"For your safety, let me check your armband and your chart to make sure everything is accurate."

add to the patient's perception that the provider "cares about the patient as a person," which is true for most providers but is not always apparent in their language. Because caring about the patient as a person is a specific question on most surveys, consistently using scripted language to convey that caring sentiment translates to high patient satisfaction scores on that measure.

Finally, language that effectively addresses specific points of patients' concern helps confirm for the patient that your staff are in tune with his needs. Any time a staff member addresses a specific area of patient concern, she is opening up the opportunity for the patient to reflect his satisfaction in the customer survey. In the

"Script Examples" section that follows, we provide a number of sample scripts that exemplify each component area, organized by specific patient concern, as well as examples of other types of scripts.

SCRIPT EXAMPLES

Addressing Specific Areas of Patient Concern

Privacy
Concern for patient privacy and discreet communication have been hallmarks of A-Team members long before the safeguards were mandated by the Health Insurance Portability and Accountability Act and institutional compliance programs. To address patient privacy, providers typically close curtains or doors and, when appropriate, lower their voices. While the provider understands that what he is doing helps ensure privacy, the patient is often unaware of this important action, and the sincere and effective effort goes unrecognized. Surprisingly, patients may give low scores for privacy even though privacy was effectively addressed. To ensure that the patient recognizes that privacy is being addressed, the provider can simply let the patient know, as we mention earlier:

"I am closing the curtain because your privacy is important to me."

"I am closing the door to give you privacy."

"I am very sorry you are in the hallway. We will get you into a more private setting as quickly as possible."

You can also give the patient choices with regard to privacy. One of us once asked a spry 88-year-old gentleman, "Shall I close this curtain for your privacy?" He said, "No, Doc, I would rather watch the show!"

Comfort
Hospitals and healthcare environments are notoriously uncomfortable, although many systems are aggressively addressing this issue. Patients, ill and often in pain, are put in rooms that are small and too cold (or warm); placed on gurneys, beds, or examining tables that are uncomfortable and place the patient in an awkward position; and given food that is often tasteless. We ask patients to undress and put

on gowns that are unflattering at best and humiliating at worst. In addition, much of what providers do causes additional discomfort and pain.

Thus, it is no surprise that surveys are created to identify concern that providers have for patients' comfort. Each staff member's efforts to address patient comfort can change patients' perception from "feeling like a number" to recognizing that the staff actually care about them. Many phrases can be adapted in script form to demonstrate concern for comfort:

"I am concerned about your comfort. May I get you a warm blanket?"

"Is there anything I can do to make you more comfortable?"

"What height shall I put the head of your bed so that you will be most comfortable?"

Delay in Initial Care

According to psychologist David Maister (1985), periods of waiting that occur *before* the service begins feel longer and create more anxiety than delays that occur after the service has started. Simply acknowledging the patient's wait can have an appeasing effect:

"I'm sorry that you've had to wait, but I'm here to take care of you now and I'm focused on your care."

Patients who have to wait become frustrated. Frustrated people often look for someone to blame, but a gentle apology can assuage that anger, particularly by emphasizing that you are now focused on them. We discuss waiting in detail in Chapter 15.

Anxiety

Generally, patients don't know precisely what to expect during their visit, which increases their anxiety and magnifies their pain. Even with scheduled appointments, the experience is often a disruptive influence on patients' and families' lives. A healthcare appointment usually requires the patient—and sometimes a family member or friend—to take time from work or the normal schedule. ED visits are even more disruptive in that patients don't expect to need them and their routines are interrupted, often in a dramatic manner. As we always tell our team, "No one wakes up in the morning and says to himself, 'What a great day! I think I'll go to the ED!'"

Even the most minor ED visits involve some degree of anxiety, and it is wise to address this emotion prospectively by acknowledging the issue and then reassuring the patient. This practice is part of the first Survival Skill core competency—making the customer service diagnosis and offering the right treatment. Most patients with chest pain are worried about a heart attack, just as patients with abdominal pain are concerned about appendicitis or—even worse—cancer.

The best way to address patients' anxiety is with effective language, as in the examples that follow:

Initial acknowledgment:

"I'm sorry this happened to you . . ."

"That sounds like it would be scary to have that happen . . ."

"While you do have chest pain . . ."

Followed by a reassuring statement:

". . . but we handle cases like yours all the time, and we will give you the best possible care."

". . . but I am glad I'm here to take care of you. You will get excellent care by our team."

". . . fortunately, your EKG and blood work tell us it is not a heart attack."

Informing About Treatment Delays

Despite the best efforts of ED providers, the multitude of processes involved in patient management simply take longer to complete than anyone desires. Patients often don't understand the details of these operational processes and perceive them as delays.

Because perceived delays in care can be the most frustrating part of the ED visit for patients, most surveys ask if patients were informed about delays. Using the same theories described above, it is important to inform patients about delays and to do so in a way that allows them to recognize that they are being informed about delays, perhaps by using those precise words. It is not ideal to say:

"We're still waiting for your laboratory test. They always do this to us. Do you have any questions?"

It is substantially more effective to say:

> "It's *important* to *me* that *you* are kept *informed* (about delays). We're still waiting for your laboratory test, but we've called to make sure it is expedited. Do you have any questions?"

A three-part approach for keeping patients informed, presented in the "Informing about treatment delays" portion of Exhibit 12.2, includes the patient satisfaction principle from the open-book test mind-set, the reason for the script, and the script itself. We have found that, if adopted, the approach almost always leads to a score of 5 by the patient.

Pain

The vast majority of patients who come to an ED have a complaint that involves pain and discomfort. Patients have an innate expectation that their complaint will be addressed. For some patients, the expectation of pain management is unrealistic:

- "Once I am evaluated, they'll give me something that takes away my pain."
- "The ED will give me whatever I want to ease my discomfort."

While healthcare providers should be experts at addressing patients' expectations related to pain as well as managing pain clinically, unfortunately, many are trained in the latter but not the former. Even worse, some providers take offense when patients have specific requests for or expectations of pain management. This scenario is complicated by the fact that many of the procedures we perform and the healing process itself involve some level of pain to get the patient to the best level of functioning. As an excellent physical therapist once said, "My job is to briefly make patients uncomfortable so they can be *really* comfortable for the long term." While it may be inappropriate or unrealistic to entirely meet patients' expectations of complete pain relief, it is always appropriate to address those expectations. To avoid the negative consequences of denying a patient's request, a provider may simply respond:

> "Yes, it is important to me that your pain is addressed. That said, I may not be able to take away your pain completely. Let's discuss it."

> "Part of the process of healing after your joint replacement is working through the discomfort that is a natural part of regaining motion and flexibility."

This acknowledgment neither implies that the provider will acquiesce to any demand nor creates an unrealistic promise that the pain will be completely eliminated or resolved.

Chronic Pain

A common and difficult problem relates to the care of the chronic pain patient. While there are actually relatively few chronic pain patients, the difficulty of managing these patients creates the perception that there are many more. When queried about the percentage of patients who inappropriately seek medication for chronic pain, it is common for groups of ED providers to estimate between 30 and 50 percent. Of course, this is nowhere near the actual percentage of chronic pain patients seen, which is less than 5 percent of total ED patients (Mayer et al. 2014), but it does reflect the level of frustration—led by lack of training—that most team members experience in managing these patients.

When attending to such patients, the following script can be very helpful:

> "I am sorry you have chronic pain. None of us can imagine how that must feel. I'm also sorry that your doctors haven't been able to manage your pain. In the emergency department, we deal with acute pain every day, but we are neither experts at managing nor qualified to manage chronic pain on an ongoing basis. I will coordinate your care with our pain management team, because its members are specifically trained and best qualified to care for your chronic pain needs."

Finally, when working with your team to develop A-Team scripts for chronic pain patients, ask them this:

> "Have you ever thought what it must be like to wake up every morning and have your first thought be, 'I'm in pain'? How would it be to go to sleep each night and think, 'It hurts'? Would *you* want that life? Neither do our patients—but that's the life they live."

Courtesy

Courtesy counts in healthcare. If you asked your grandmother or another elderly relative, "What is the most important characteristic in a doctor or nurse?" the most common answer would be, "Good bedside manners!" In 2008, the American Board of Medical Specialties performed just such a survey, with this result: "95 percent of participants surveyed said that bedside manner and communications skills are very important or important as a key factor when choosing a doctor."

Consider the alternate approach, sometimes sarcastically described as, "I'm here to save your life, not fluff your pillow" or with other, even less polite, words. (Remember the T-shirts we bought for our nurses?) Patients arrive fearful, in pain, vulnerable. Then their clothes are taken away and they are placed in an uncomfortable room and have multiple personnel come and go with no regard for their privacy. Worse, patients may undergo painful procedures. If the patient's dignity is taken away by rude, sarcastic, and uncaring staff, the providers are literally adding insult to injury. It is no wonder that surveys ask about the courteousness of the providers. Earlier in the book we suggest some ways to promote a culture of courtesy, but suffice to say here that it always helps to remind the team that a healthy dose of "Ma'ams" and "Sirs" goes a long way with our patients and their families, not to mention the others who observe us when we are "onstage."

Active and Effective Listening

We discuss in Chapter 7 the importance of being a trained and skilled listener, but it deserves repeating that listening well

- improves relationships,
- exhibits sincerity,
- enhances understanding,
- decreases misunderstanding, and
- promotes cooperation.

Some basic scripts help capture this behavior.

"I'm going to sit here so that I can listen carefully to you."

"It's important to me that I listen to what you have to say."

"If I heard you correctly, you said that . . ."

"I want to make sure we understand what you are saying."

"Let me close this door so we aren't distracted when we talk."

"I apologize for having to take this phone call, but I want to get right back to what you were saying when I come back."

These phrases don't have to be followed verbatim, and the team will want to add their own "signature" to the precise wording.

Additional Examples

Many examples of scripts have been devised by others, all with the goal of improving the communication between and perceptions of the patients/families and caregivers.

Scripts, Scribes, and the Electronic Medical Record

Virtually all hospitals use electronic medical records (EMRs) or are in the process of phasing them in. Scripts play an important part in ensuring that patients understand what the EMR is for and the reasons we need to spend time with the computer as well as the patient. If we don't use scripts, patients will predictably think that clinicians are on the computer for reasons that have nothing to do with patient care.

One of the best flow-related solutions to dealing with EMRs is using scribes—typically college students with an interest in the health professions—who follow the physicians and nurses and record the clinician–patient interactions into the EMR. Of course, they do not perform computerized provider order entry (CPOE), but they represent an effective way to maximize the time physicians and nurses spend interacting directly with the patient.

Here are examples of how scripts can work, with and without scribes.

With scribes:

"This is Liza, who is one of our scribes. She is working with me to ensure that we accurately capture all of your pertinent information on your computerized medical record. This process is both for accuracy and for your safety."

Without scribes:

"Now that I have all of your initial information, I will be spending some time on the computer to make sure we document this information in the computerized medical record. This process is both for accuracy and for your safety."

Creating Previews and Expectations

Two areas in which scripts can be particularly helpful are

1. creating previews (a sense of what will happen to the patient during her visit) and
2. creating expectations (a sense of how much time the patient should expect to spend—which you can aim to exceed).

Following are some examples of preview-building and expectation-managing scripts in healthcare:

"Do you have any questions? I have plenty of time."

"I'm Dr. Maguire, and your nurse and I are leading an excellent team that will be caring for you."

"Even when we're not in the room, we're still guiding your care."

"I'm sorry this happened to you."

"Come back any time; we never close."

"Thank you for allowing us to take care of you."

"I must leave to respond to a call. I will try to be back in 20 minutes" (expecting that you will actually be back in 5 minutes).

We've written previously about expectation creation and using this tool to make time work for us by providing previews by which we wisely overestimate the time it will take us to deliver on a promise, just as The Walt Disney Company teaches its staff. In the example above, using the theory of (exaggerated) expectation setting, the provider set an expectation with the patient of returning in 20 minutes. He had expected to take only 5 minutes but was actually away from the patient for 15 minutes. By creating an exaggerated time expectation, however, the provider, who returned later than he expected, still was back with the patient in less time than the patient expected.

Pauze's Pearls

The best scripts are those the team members devise themselves, in part because staff are most likely to put them into practice on a daily basis in the course of their work. For example, Denis Pauze, MD, an ED physician at our hospital, devised the following scripts (aka Pauze's Pearls) to help communicate more effectively with the patients he saw on the night shift (Pauze 2011):

"I'm going to be here all night. If you have any questions, give me a call."

"I'll be on duty Tuesday and Wednesday nights. If you need to see me, come back then."

"You've already had to wait tonight. If you come back Tuesday or Wednesday, give this card to the triage nurse, and I'll see you in the triage area as soon as I can."

This set of scripts is an excellent example of using your service champions' insights for the benefit of all your patients and all your staff. *We* didn't come up with Pauze's Pearls—Denis did. But we *did* create a culture and an environment where *all* team members felt empowered to create scripts that make their jobs easier—and the patients' lives better. You should, too.

SURVIVAL SKILLS SUMMARY

- All language has meaning. Make your language work for you and your patients.
- Scripts avoid the "law of unintended consequences" and help predictably ensure that our communication is understood as we meant it to be.
- Scripts are evidence-based language that taps into what works from the A-Team's experience.
- Scripts should also be survey based, in that they should be tied to what specifically is being measured by the survey questions.
- When resistance is encountered, remind staff that scripts are the ACLS, the ATLS, and the core measures of communication.
- Use scripts to maximize the ROI on a precious resource—your time.
- Make scripts personal (*I/We,* not *They/Those guys*).
- The team should always help devise the scripts (remember Pauze's Pearls).
- As a leader, you *must* create the culture of empowerment so your A-Team members feel comfortable sharing their scripts.

NOTE

1. The general concept of putting language to work to serve our patients' needs—and to make our jobs easier—which we refer to as a combined EBL–SBL approach, is essentially the same as what the Studer Group calls Key Words at Key Times, although they were developed independently (Studer 2014). In addition, many insights from our great friend Dr. Rob Strauss are reflected in this chapter (Strauss and Mayer 2014).

REFERENCES

American Board of Medical Specialties. 2008. "Facts About the 2008 ABMS Consumer Survey: How Americans Choose Their Doctors." Press release. www.abms.org/News_and_Events/Media_Newsroom/pdf/ABMS_Survey_Fact_Sheet.pdf.

Maister, D. 1985. "The Psychology of Waiting Lines." In *The Service Encounter*, edited by J. A. Czepiel, M. R. Solomon, and C. Suprenant. Lanham, MD: Lexington Books.

Mayer, T. A., J. Kaplan, R. W. Strauss, and R. J. Cates. 2014. "Customer Service in Emergency Medicine." In *Strauss and Mayer's Emergency Department Management*, edited by R. W. Strauss and T. A. Mayer. New York: McGraw-Hill.

Merton, R. K. 1936. "The Unintended Consequences of Purposive Social Action." *American Sociological Review* 1 (6): 894–904.

Pauze, D. 2011. Personal communication, March 14.

CHAPTER 13

A-Team Tool 6—Hiring Right

When you consider Carlzon's (1987) "moments of truth" insight in terms of creating and sustaining a culture of service excellence, you are led to an inexorable conclusion:

The hiring of a new employee may be the most expensive decision you ever make.

Because the people delivering the service define the hospital and healthcare system, the process of hiring, selecting, onboarding, and coaching those people is an essential part of our jobs. We believe that you must hire right for customer service—that you must screen for the customer service gene. How often is that belief evident in the hiring practices at your hospital? Is customer service a part of the interview process? Most of us say "yes," but there is usually a disconnect between our words and our actions.

Are the hirings at your facility contingent on the results of a customer service evaluation? Are the following questions asked of potential employees?

◆ Have you ever had a patient who was really angry? How did you deal with that?
◆ When you have patients with unreasonable expectations, what do you say to them?
◆ How do you handle patients who complain to you?
◆ If one of your direct reports tells you she has "had it with all the complainers," what advice do you give her?
◆ Tell me about a time you felt really great about the service you provided to a patient.
◆ What are you *most* proud of in your career?
◆ What are you *least* proud of?

- Tell me about a time you broke the rules on behalf of better patient care?
- Who are your mentors, and why?
- When you are working with a B-Team member, how do you let him know his actions aren't helping?

If we are going to screen for the customer service gene, we need to add a couple of important items to the above questions we are asking when we interview people. Two of the best questions for hiring physicians are:

1. What is the worst thing I'm going to hear about you?
2. Who am I going to hear it from?

You can also ask their previous supervisor:

- How does this person make other people feel?
- When you see this person's name on the schedule, how does your staff react? With smiles? Or do they poke their eyes out and run in the other direction?

GUIDELINES FOR HIRING RIGHT

Hiring for Qualities as Well as for Qualifications

These questions translate to the central focus of hiring right: to check the *qualities* as closely as you check the *qualifications*. The table that follows specifies how these characteristics should be evaluated:

Qualifications	Qualities
Employer	Employees
College(s)	Colleagues
Honors	Honor
Education	Ethics
Aptitude	Attitude
Degree(s)	Demeanor
Credentials	Credibility
Intelligence	Integrity
Computer skills	Customer skills

When you hire staff, you check with their colleges, but do you check with their colleagues? The curriculum vitae tells you if they received honors, but do they have honor? Their education is apparent for all to see, but what about their ethics? Their transcripts and job evaluations can tell you about their intelligence, but shouldn't you also ask about their integrity? Hiring right requires that you pay attention to *both* columns. Think about this—if you had to change the attributes in one column versus the other, which would be easier to change? Without question, the attributes in the "Qualities" column are far more difficult, perhaps impossible, to change.

You can train people, you can send them back to school, you can give them technical skills, and you can improve their qualifications. But if you have a "qualities loser," you most likely have a loser for life. Regardless of how tough hiring is, regardless of the shortage of workers, stay away from qualities losers. Why? *It only takes one B-Team member to destroy an entire shift.* The impact that hiring a qualities loser—someone who lacks the positive characteristics listed in the right-hand column of that table—has on morale is devastating. At BestPractices, our physician application requires that each applicant list three patients and three nurses we can call as customer service references.

Equally important is the impact that your hiring decision will have on future hiring decisions:

A-Team members hire A-Team members.
B-Team members hire C-Team members.

A-Team members always seek to surround themselves with excellence. They know that truly great leaders hire people who can perform equally to or even outperform the leaders in a given area. And the team is made stronger for these skills, especially when those skills are superior. That is how an organization improves.

B-Team members, on the other hand, always feel in competition with their own team members, in part because of their fundamental feelings of inadequacy. So instead of hiring someone at their own perceived level of competence, they hire someone *below* that level—a C-Team member—who will not challenge them. This is a doubly bankrupt strategy: Not only are they hiring down but their own feelings of inadequacy cause them to underestimate their own true potential.

Supporting That New Hire

Hiring right also means onboarding and orienting for service excellence. If staff hear all about the importance of service to the culture of the organization, yet the orientation lacks any substantive material on the subject, they will know that there is a disconnect between what was sold to them and what the organization truly values. Take a close look at your orientation and onboarding process for all team members—particularly for physicians. Does it truly reflect the mission, vision, and values you have so carefully crafted and communicated? Or is it full of meaningless information? We actually know of one CEO who, in an *Undercover Boss* move, attended all the orientation sessions for new physicians. She was shocked at what she found and immediately overhauled the entire process. There had been a complete disconnect in what was being said by people who had basically been "reading from a script" of inane promises being made to new physicians, which had no passion and no connection to the primary purpose of "Patient First." She personally assured staff that the message was one of "making promises we not only can, but will, keep each day, every day." Those promises were focused on honesty; transparency; connection to the mission, vision, and values of the institution; and an open-door policy of all senior leadership team members to answer physicians' questions or concerns. Physician loyalty scores predictably rose and have been sustained over time.

Re-recruiting the A-Team

Of course, hiring right and "onboarding right" aren't the entire process. New staff should undergo 30-, 60-, and 90-day appraisals of how they are acting on the words they told us during the interview process. Naturally, this assessment will include clinical competence issues, but it should also include rescreening for the customer service gene. Do the words and music match with this physician or employee? If not, leaders must hold them accountable for their actions and the perceptions thereof.

Furthermore, we believe that ongoing accountability has to include rescreening for service excellence and all A-Team behaviors. In this way, we can constantly re-recruit our A-Team members by giving them positive feedback (see Chapter 16, "Rewarding Champions") and periodically asking them, "Are we still meeting your career needs? What would you like to see more/less of?" Finally, use your A-Team members as coaches and mentors for B-Team members.

CONCLUSION

Hiring right, onboarding right, and re-recruiting your A-Team members are the foundation of a highly motivated and empowered team. Without these processes, service excellence is rare, and when it does occur, it is an accident, not a logical consequence of the organization's culture and structure.

SURVIVAL SKILLS SUMMARY

◆ The hiring of a new employee or physician is one of the most crucial and, ultimately, most expensive decisions a leader will ever make.
◆ Screen for the customer service gene in all hiring decisions.
◆ Ask probing questions to help you glean examples of prospective hires' service commitment.
◆ Screen for both qualities and qualifications.
◆ If you hire a "qualities loser," you have probably hired a loser for life.
◆ A-Team members hire A-Team members. B-Team members hire C-Team members.
◆ Hiring right is important, but so is onboarding right.
◆ Continue to hold staff accountable after they have been hired and onboarded by using frequent evaluations to rescreen for the customer service gene.
◆ Continue to re-recruit your A-Team members and use them as coaches and mentors.

REFERENCE

Carlzon, J. 1987. *Moments of Truth: New Strategies for Today's Customer-Driven Economy*. New York: HarperCollins.

MORE RESOURCES ON HIRING RIGHT

Block, P. 2002. *The Answer to How Is Yes*. San Francisco: Berrett-Koehler.

A truly inspirational book from one of the most incisive minds writing about leadership.

Greenleaf, R. K. 2002. *Servant Leadership: A Journey into the Nature of Legitimate Power and Greatness.* New York: Paulist Press.

A collection of essays defining servant leadership, including Greenleaf's seminal essay launching the concept of servant leadership. Essays by Stephen Covey and Peter Senge are also excellent.

Kotter, J. P. 1996. *Leading Change.* Boston: Harvard Business School Press.

The definitive text on change management, an essential tool for any service excellence initiative.

Press, I. 2002. *Patient Satisfaction: Defining, Measuring, and Improving the Experience of Care.* Chicago: Health Administration Press.

A scholarly and detailed approach from the nation's éminence grise *in patient satisfaction surveys—and a great friend.*

Sanders, B. 1995. *Fabled Service: Ordinary Acts, Extraordinary Outcomes.* San Diego: Pfieffer.

A fast but good read, blending elements of the Nordstrom philosophy with great insights and quotes from Tom Peters, Sam Wattson, Jan Carlzon, and Mother Teresa.

Connellan, T. 1997. *Inside the Magic Kingdom: Seven Keys to Disney's Success.* Austin, TX: Bard Press.

Spector, R., and P. McCarthy. 1995. *The Nordstrom Way.* New York: John Wiley.

Two brief books with insights from two service industry leaders.

CHAPTER 14

A-Team Tool 7—Innovation:
Next-Level Thinking

While all of the A-Team Tool Kit's elements are important, perhaps the least intuitive, and therefore most important to discuss, is the leverage we can afford our teams by focusing on our accomplishments and taking them to the next level. When we look at our customer service scores and see the progress we have made (and, more importantly, how we have *made our jobs easier* along the way), we often find ourselves still short of the targets we have set. Even worse are the situations where the scores are perpetual "cellar dwellers"—and seem to be going further south. The A-Team Tool discussed in this chapter can help us to reach our targets and ensure that we are not heading in the wrong direction instead.

We start with the landmark work of Jim Collins. In a series of books that includes *Built to Last* (Collins and Porras 1994), *Good to Great* (Collins 2001), and *Great by Choice* (Collins and Hansen 2011), Collins has done a great service to all who work in healthcare by noting that, of all the institutions that achieve high levels of success, far fewer are able to make the leap to greatness (Collins 2001). His detailed and elegant matched-pair study of successful companies shows that there is an inflection point at which great companies are able to accelerate the pace of transformational change to an entirely different and more sustainable level (Exhibit 14.1). Knowing this inflection point and knowing *what to do* at that time is one of the most important things that healthcare leaders can do to go "from good to great." First, though, we must focus on the "why"—why we want or need to improve. Then, and only then, do we focus on "how."

Exhibit 14.1: The Good-to-Great Matched-Pair Research Method

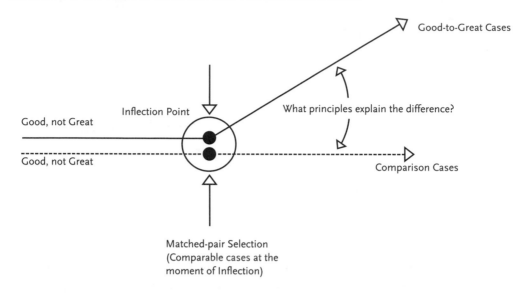

Source: Reproduced with permission from "Where are you on your journey from Good to Great? Good to Great® Diagnostic Tool." www.jimcollins.com/tools/diagnostic-tool.pdf.

WHY IMPROVE?

It's clear that a key strategy is knowing how to notice when we are at that inflection point and what to do when we find ourselves there. Less clear are the facts that underlie the inflection point and precisely how to leverage progress at that point. Whether it is the cellar-dwelling dilemma ("How do we move from 'worst' to 'first'?") or the good-to-great conundrum ("We've reached the 75th percentile on our scores, but the 90th percentile is our target"), we have to start with destroying one of the most pervasive and pernicious myths in all of healthcare, which is this:

You want us to go from good to great, but it is all those complainers and crusaders, who give us scores of 1 or 2, who are killing us and keeping us from making more progress. You can never please some people!

All of us have heard this lament from some of our leaders, managers, and team members at one time or another—usually just after the disappointing scores have been posted. We call this "the myth of the low-lie-ers" or "myth of the miscreants." However—and it is impossible to overstate the importance of this—*not only is the myth false but it is demonstrably false on a statistical basis.* Analysis we have conducted of data from virtually every survey, including HCAHPS scores, demonstrates irrefutably that the myth of the low-lie-ers is simply that—a myth. Exhibits 14.2 and 14.3 show data from the two largest survey companies, PRC and Press Ganey, respectively, that reveal the lie to this myth.

Let's start with destroying the myth. Look carefully at the bottom line of Exhibit 14.3, showing a team at the 35th percentile. It's easy to imagine the team bemoaning that it's impossible to go from worst to first and that it is the low-lie-ers who are holding them back. But look closely at the data. The difference between the percentage of patients giving them a 1 on the scale is only one point higher for the 35th percentile team than the 99th percentile team! And the 2s are the same.

Similarly, if we look back at Exhibit 14.2, derived from PRC's national database, if half of the patients currently rating us as a 4 ("very good") instead rated us as a 5 ("excellent"), we would move from merely average to near the top five hospitals in the United States on this measure.

The leverage for progress is "taking 4s to 5s," by which we mean that our real focus shouldn't be on the lower side of the scales but on getting people who are already giving us a score of "very good" to give us a score of "excellent." If we can

Exhibit 14.2: Measures of Overall Care Quality, 2013

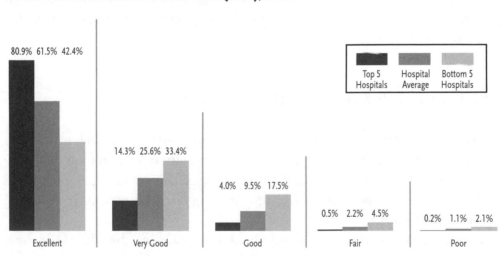

Source: Data from PRC National Inpatient Database, 2013, "Overall Quality of Care."

Exhibit 14.3: Taking 4s to 5s

	1s	2s	3s	4s	5s
99th Percentile Hospital	1%	2%	7%	24%	66%
64th Percentile Hospital	1%	2%	8%	34%	55%
35th Percentile Hospital	2%	2%	8%	36%	52%

Source: Data from Press Ganey, March 2007.

bring those "good" people, whose expectations we feel we are exceeding, to give us an "excellent," we will seriously move the needle in the right direction. In fact, it only takes about one-third of those ranking us as "good" to rank us as "great" or "excellent" for us to move from the 35th percentile to nearly the 99th percentile. That's the leverage of going from good to great, or in the language of surveys, "very good to excellent."

We cannot hope to make progress in accelerating the pace of change unless and until we burst this myth. The myth is paralyzing to progress precisely because it distracts us from focusing on high scores and instead focusing on the low scores, since taking the 4s to 5s is the real issue.

The Influence of Six Sigma on Healthcare Service

As you recall, we have constantly reiterated that our primary focus in our work has not been on raising scores per se, but rather in accentuating A-Team tools that *make our jobs easier.* Are we reneging on this with our emphasis on taking 4s to 5s? Not at all. Going from good to great is simply making our jobs *even easier* by taking improvement to the next level.

The same principle applies to 4-point Likert scales or the HCAHPS scale of "always, usually, sometimes, never." Predictably, the ability to make progress depends on those who already are giving us credit, but they need to give us a little more credit, which affords us a place where applying the lessons of Six Sigma can provide leverage to subtly encourage them to do so.

The precepts of Six Sigma were first used in the United States by Motorola and General Electric to dramatically increase the yield of defect-free manufacturing. (For an engaging and helpful explanation of Six Sigma and its application in healthcare, see Barry, Murcko, and Brubaker 2002.) Virginia Mason Medical Center in Seattle used Six Sigma in much of its original work to develop its Virginia Mason Production System by which to improve the reliability of healthcare (VMMC 2014).

The graph in Exhibit 14.4 shows how an organization can use the tools and culture of Six Sigma to march from the large number of defects at the bottom left of the graph (with a wide skew of variability and 308,540 defects per million) to the desired state of few defects on the upper right (with a very narrow skew and only 3.4 defects per million, or six sigma). In other words, as the number of defects in a product or service is reduced, the skew of the results "tightens" considerably.

In the case of patient satisfaction data, as more and more patients rate your care as "very good," or a 4, or as "excellent," a 5, the narrower the skew of the scores becomes. The practical result of these data trending toward higher scores is that small changes in patient satisfaction raw scores necessarily result in dramatic increases in percentile rankings, as we show in exhibits 14.2 and 14.3.

Specifically, look at the breakout of scores in exhibits 14.2 and 14.3 and compare them with Exhibit 14.4, which shows the narrowing of the skew as progress occurs. You should come to the same conclusion we have regarding healthcare patient satisfaction scores: We are already approaching a rate of defects equal to six sigma, since the majority of the scores are 4s and 5s. The skew of the scores in exhibits 14.2 and 14.3 is very narrow to begin with, so either going from worst to first or from average to being ranked a top-five hospital does not require a massive shift of opinion. But it does require a laser focus on taking 4s to 5s to move from good to great.

As we do so, it is important to remember the wisdom of Tom Peters, who said:

> If you're getting better, but your competition is getting better faster—you are getting worse!

So that's the "why." Now let's look at the "how." At the considerable risk of exhibiting some hubris, much of the "how" is in applying elements of the A-Team Tool Kit to the good-to-great dilemma.

Exhibit 14.4: Example of Six Sigma Improvement Metrics

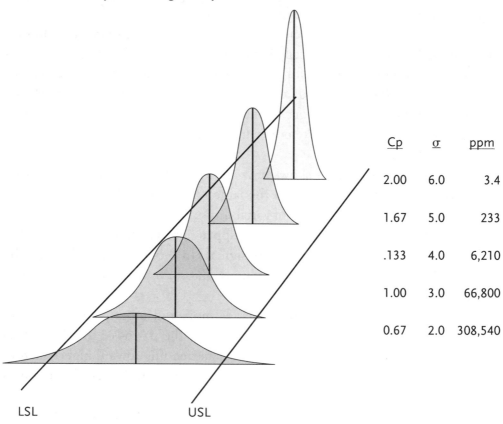

Cp	σ	ppm
2.00	6.0	3.4
1.67	5.0	233
.133	4.0	6,210
1.00	3.0	66,800
0.67	2.0	308,540

Note: LSL = lower specification limit; USL = upper specification limit; Cp = process capability; ppm = parts per million.

HOW TO IMPROVE

Consider the following simple example demonstrating how we might apply particular A-Team behaviors and A-Team Tool Kit skills to the HCAHPS survey question concerning the ability of the doctor or nurse to explain to the patient the results of his care and tests:

During this hospital stay, how often did the doctors/nurses explain things to you in a way you could understand?

Applicable A-Team Behaviors

- **Sit down.** The patient will perceive the doctor is in the room three to five times longer than if she were to stand, potentially exceeding the patient's expectations related to the length of the visit.
- **Active listening.** Exhibiting this behavior increases the accuracy of information exchange and makes the patient a part of the process by restating what the doctor has said. It also ensures that the patient's expectations are clearly understood and that both the customer service diagnosis and clinical diagnosis are addressed.
- **Blameless apology.** "I am so sorry I didn't explain this more clearly, but let's take the time to do so now" is an example of using the blameless apology to great effect.

Applicable A-Team Tools

- **Empowerment—point-of-impact intervention** allows the doctor to correct misunderstandings of explanations at the time they occur.
- **Empowerment—service recovery** allows physicians to correct errors or misunderstandings of care and tests as rapidly as possible.
- **Empowerment—leading up** makes other members of the team a part of the ongoing explanation of tests and care.
- **Focused patient satisfaction coaching** allows trending of data from scores on explanation by specific physician and by reporting period to coach and mentor to A-Team actions that are more effective. For example, "Dr. Roberts, your scores on ability to effectively explain care to patients and their families continues to trend downward. We will be having you work with Dr. Alleva, who has 99th percentile scores and will coach you on how she does it."
- **Rounding** puts leaders in a position to identify both problems and A-Team explanation processes on a real-time basis. Sign-out and bedside rounding provide fail-safe approaches to explaining findings and answering questions. Whiteboards offer a means of further ensuring the foolproof transmission of information. Rounding on next uses patient callbacks to ask patients who ranked us as a 4, "What could we have done to merit a 5?" Similarly, it allows the organization to ask those who gave it a 5, "What *specifically* was done that made you feel we provided excellent care?"
- **Scripts** provide a template for consistently excellent communications with patients. For example, "It's important to me that I take the *time* to *explain the results of your tests and the progress of your care.* Please let me know if you have any questions about this."

- **Hiring right** ensures that the ability to explain in clear and succinct terms is part of the hiring, orientation, and mentoring processes.
- **Moving 4s to 5s** focuses on the 4s to move about a third of them to 5s using all the tools listed here.
- **Flow** is a means by which to build explanations into the process of designing flow efforts into the system, for example, ensuring that CT scan results are called in or e-mailed to the physician so she can get the results to the patient as rapidly as possible.

Each of these tools has an impact on our ability to leverage 4s to 5s in this instance. Taken together, they put us in a much stronger position to attain our goal of making the job *even* easier and moving the needle from good to great.

Of course, as leaders we will deal with the B-Team members and their behaviors that lead to scores in the 1, 2, or 3 range. But the most important leverage is on the other end of the scale, and we should invest time in leading our team from very good to excellent.

SURVIVAL SKILLS SUMMARY

- Advancing to the highest levels of healthcare service requires application of the A-Team tools that involve taking 4s to 5s, or moving from good to great.
- The inflection point from good to great must be recognized, as well as what to do once we get there.
- Taking 4s to 5s means making our jobs *even easier.*
- The myth of the miscreants or low-lie-ers is that those who are giving us low scores (1, 2, or 3) are "killing us."
- Unless and until the myth is busted, we can't progress to the highest levels of customer service and patient satisfaction.
- The skew in healthcare customer service scores is extremely narrow. Small changes in scores result in dramatic increases in percentile rankings.
- If we can leverage approximately one-third of people who say we are "good" (a score of 4) to say we are "great" or "excellent" (a score of 5), we can dramatically improve patients' ratings of our care.
- The above goal is best accomplished by using the three A-Team behaviors and the nine A-Team Tool Kit elements described in the example used in this chapter.

REFERENCES

Barry, R., A. C. Murcko, and C. Brubaker. 2002. *The Six Sigma Book for Healthcare: Improving Outcomes by Reducing Errors.* Chicago: Health Administration Press.

Collins, J. 2001. *Good to Great: Why Some Companies Make the Leap . . . and Others Don't.* New York: Harper Business.

Collins, J., and M. T. Hansen. 2011. *Great by Choice: Uncertainty, Chaos, and Luck.* New York: HarperCollins.

Collins, J., and J. Porras. 1994. *Built to Last: Successful Habits of Visionary Companies.* New York: HarperCollins.

Virginia Mason Medical Center (VMMC). 2014. "Virginia Mason Production System." www.virginiamason.org/VMPS.

CHAPTER 15

A-Team Tool 8—Flow and the Psychology of Waiting

We live in interesting times. The capacity-constrained environments in which we work require us to find creative and sustainable ways to become *the high-quality, low-cost providers* of care while simultaneously ensuring that safety, reliability, risk reduction, and service are not eroded. It's quite a challenge, because it means we are essentially being asked to do more with less (IHI 2005). Along with our colleague and friend Dr. Kirk Jensen, we have written a great deal elsewhere about flow across the dimensions of healthcare (Jensen et al. 2007; Mayer and Jensen 2009, 2012), and we discuss a number of those key points here.

DEFINING FLOW

We can't improve flow if we can't define it. Our definition of flow is as follows:

> Flow exists to the extent that we *add value* and *decrease waste* by increasing benefits and decreasing burdens as our patients move through the service transitions and queues of healthcare.

We clearly have a Lean focus in how we define flow in that we use Lean's language of adding value and eliminating waste. We do so to help emphasize the need for both leaders and bedside clinicians to find creative ways to increase value and eliminate any activity that doesn't add value (waste).

Value can be defined on the macroeconomic level or at the level of bedside providers. At the macroeconomic level of healthcare planning, Porter and Lee (2013) define value as a ratio of healthcare outcomes divided by the cost to provide those outcomes:

$$\text{Value} = \frac{\text{Outcomes}}{\text{Cost}}$$

While this definition is important in the broad debate on value, it is of limited help to clinicians and leaders as they deal with patients. Porter (2010) himself notes:

> Value measurement in healthcare today is limited and highly imperfect. Not only is outcome data lacking, but understanding of the true costs of care is virtually absent.

Donald J. Berwick, MD, former CEO of IHI, adds, "When it comes to healthcare value, we are in measurement adolescence" (Berwick and Hackbarth 2012).

In light of these limitations, we have worked with our friend and colleague Len Berry and others to define value for bedside providers in a more pragmatic way by this calculus (Mayer and Jensen 2009; Toussaint and Berry 2013):

$$\text{Value} = \frac{\text{Benefits received}}{\text{Burdens endured}}$$

We have found that this definition is one that physicians and nurses understand intuitively and embrace enthusiastically. Following is a simple example from the ED that shows how this definition can be put to work.

The most common presenting symptom in the ED is abdominal pain. How do we add value and eliminate waste by increasing benefits and decreasing burdens for patients who present with abdominal pain? Some benefits from treatment in the ED that occur for these patients are

- pain relief,
- hydration,
- nausea treatment,
- getting an accurate diagnosis, and
- reassurance that "it's not serious."

The burdens endured by these patients include

- the time it takes to get the studies done and medications administered,
- pain from blood draws or IV starts,
- side effects of medicines, and
- the inconvenience of drinking oral contrast solutions.

If we can increase benefits *and* decrease burdens, we will have added value and diminished waste. How does that work? Using our abdominal pain example, here are some ways to add value by increasing benefits:

Category	Flow Action
Pain relief	Pain protocols, rapid-acting agents
Hydration	Rapid IV access, fluid bolus, use of IV and PO routes
Nausea treatment	Rapid IV medications
Accurate diagnosis	Imaging protocols, evidence-based medicine (EBM)–guided workup
Reassurance	Rapid results communicated clearly, e.g., "Good news! Your tests show no signs of cancer."

Similarly, we can improve flow by decreasing the burdens for abdominal pain patients by decreasing or eliminating unnecessary burdens.

Category	Flow Action
Time to studies/medication	Immediate pain/nausea treatment
Pain from blood draws/IVs	Topical anesthetics, IV and blood draw together
Side effects	EBM protocols, asking patients about side effects
Oral contrast	Eliminate routine use of oral contrast

THE VALUE OF FLOW

The elimination of the routine use of oral contrast in abdominal CTs affects flow in several ways: it decreases the burden of drinking the liquid, decreases length of stay by two to three hours on average, and creates (or preserves) additional capacity for other patients by eliminating the time needed for the patient to drink the liquid. For an ED with 40,000 visits performing 9,000 abdominal CTs per year (the national average), eliminating the routine use of oral contrast, which takes three hours on average, creates 27,000 hours of additional capacity for the ED. If the average length of stay for the ED is two and a half hours, this flow effort results in creating the capacity to see an additional 10,800 patients per year. If the net collected revenue per ED patient is $100 for the emergency physician and $400 for the hospital, the revenue impact of these additional patients is $1,080,000 and $4,320,000, respectively. So the financial impact of flow is considerable.

THE IMPORTANCE OF FLOW

We've talked at length about A-Team and B-Team members and their behaviors. We've also talked about A-Team and B-Team processes. In terms of flow, it is critical to understand that

A-Team members trump B-Team members, but B-Team processes can frustrate even the best of A-Team members. And if leaders allow B-Team processes to persist, it destroys the A-Team members' morale—and erodes the entire team's confidence in the leader.

In blunt terms, the importance of flow puts leaders' credibility at stake if the leaders systematically allow processes and systems to persist that do not add value and that allow waste. However, if leaders aggressively pursue flow and the value that drives it while also eliminating the waste that everyone can see, they place themselves at the inflection point that then allows their organizations to go from good to great. So, other than your credibility and your organization's future, there is not that much at stake in ignoring flow, right?! Leaders must think of accentuating value as a treasure hunt and eliminating waste as a bounty hunt.

PUTTING FLOW TO WORK

There are many examples of flow in both the ED and hospital environments, examples of which are shown here.

Emergency Department Flow Solutions

Steps for implementing flow solutions in the ED include the following:

- **Triage bypass or direct to room.** When ED rooms are available, patients are taken directly to the room after a basic "name, demographics, and chief complaint" at triage, which speeds care.
- **Advanced triage guidelines for nurses.** When all rooms are full, nurses begin testing and care through standing physician orders, such as ankle X-rays for sports injuries and urinalysis for frequency.

- **Team triage (physician or mid-level provider in triage).** When all rooms are full, and will be for an extended time, or when the number of patients predictably exceeds the number of available beds, a team composed of a physician (or mid-level provider), nurse, tech, scribe, and registrar is deployed to the triage area (Mayer 2005).
- **Results waiting room.** Patients are kept in ED rooms only as long as needed and then moved to a comfortable waiting area to await their results and discharge.
- **Fast Track.** Patients with low acuity are triaged to a specific area with specific staff to care for their needs according to evidence-based protocols.
- **Level 3 Fast Track.** Patients with higher acuity than Fast Track but unlikely to require admission are treated in an area designated for their care.

All of these ED flow solutions (discussed in more detail in Jensen et al. [2007] and Mayer and Jensen [2009, 2012]) represent ways in which the following flow principles have been made practical:

- *Triage is a process, not a place.*
- *Get the patient and the doctor together as quickly and as safely as possible.*
- Fast Track *is a verb, not a noun.*
- *We should be fast at fast things and slow at slow things.*
- *Horizontal patients value real estate (a bed); vertical patients value speed.*
- *Not all patients need a bed, and not every patient who does, needs it for the entire ED stay.*

Hospital Flow Solutions

Some of the most important and exciting work on flow has occurred on the hospital side of the equation. In that environment in particular, we have found that one of flow's biggest enemies is putting up with the status quo. When the question is asked, "Why are we doing it this way?" the most common answer is, "Because we've *always* done it this way." Increasing value and decreasing waste require a courageous leadership approach that challenges our team members to think in new and creative ways. Think for a moment about how a bed is put back in service at most hospitals:

It is 2:00 p.m. on a weekday on a medical/surgical floor. A patient has just been discharged from bed 462 on that floor. What are the steps necessary to get a different patient assigned to and into bed 462?

You will likely come up with the following steps:

1. The staff nurse or charge nurse calls environmental services (EVS) to let that department know the bed needs to be cleaned.
2. EVS assigns and informs a team member to clean bed 462.
3. The EVS team member finishes his current task and heads to 462.
4. The EVS team member cleans 462.
5. The EVS team member informs the charge nurse or staff nurse that 462 is clean.
6. The charge or staff nurse informs the bed board that 462 is available.

Now think about this—what happens at 3:00 p.m. on most medical/surgical floors? Of course, we all know it is change of shift. Now ask yourself this "flow question"—What is the incentive for the staff nurse to get that bed back in service and a new patient into it before 3 p.m.? Actually, there is a disincentive to do so, since getting a new patient is just "more work." At any good restaurant, the wait staff actually want to "turn the table" as quickly as possible, since it not only demonstrates good service but also provides a chance to increase income from tips—nurses do not have such an incentive.

Add to this the fact that most hospitals actually *decrease* the EVS staff (often by as much as one-third) at 3 p.m., and the flow impact of "because we've always done it that way" becomes apparent. "Be a Bed Ahead" programs, first used at Inova Fairfax Hospital (Mayer 2005), address this problem by preassigning beds on the basis of patient acuity and informing the charge nurse on that floor that they are next up for an admission. The charge nurse then assigns and informs the nurse on that unit with the fewest patients that she will be getting the next admission so she can plan accordingly.

Flow Solutions for Other Areas

Other hospitalwide flow solutions include the following:

♦ **Early bed decision.** Experienced emergency physicians and nurses typically can identify many, if not most, of the patients who will need admission. These patients are identified early for the admitting physician, with lab and imaging studies performed only as needed to properly identify the appropriate bed and treatment.

- **Early request for a bed.** Similar to early bed decision and Be a Bed Ahead, this step extends the concept of parallel, as opposed to sequential, processing by requesting an inpatient bed early in the course of care. This is particularly helpful in hospitals where getting a bed can take 30 minutes or longer.
- **Expedited testing.** In certain cases, diagnostic testing may explicitly determine either the need for admission or bed location, with the goal of eliminating bottlenecks and rate-limiting steps. Point-of-care (POC) testing may expedite care, as when using an EKG and POC troponin for acute chest syndrome or a portable chest X-ray, an EKG, a dip urinalysis, and POC electrolytes for many medical admissions.
- **Early notification of the admitting team.** The concept of informing the admitting team early is a powerful one and is promoted by the advent of the specialty of hospital medicine. It is very much a two-way street in that this particular culture change allows the emergency medicine and hospital medicine physicians to see inside each other's worlds. For emergency physicians and nurses, the questions that need to be answered related to potential admissions include the following:

  - Does the patient need admission? Why?
  - What service does she need to be admitted to?
  - Does that service have the right resources? Why?
  - What needs to be done *now* that will best expedite the patient's care?
  - What evidence supports all of the decisions above?

- Early notification creates an ongoing dialogue that can reap substantial benefits and creates a partnership between emergency medicine and hospital medicine.

EXPRESS ADMITTING UNITS

Many busy emergency departments have a constant stream of patients coming in, through both emergency medical services and "walk-ins." If we can't "open the back door of the ED," we can't keep the front door of the ED open. Many hospitals have addressed this situation by creating express admitting units (EAUs). These units are geographically separate from the ED and designed to give the patient a place to be held until an inpatient bed is available. It also allows the admitting team to continue evaluation and testing, which, if driven by evidence-based protocols, enhances decision making on what is the most appropriate bed and what is the most appropriate treatment.

The most important caveat when considering EAUs is that they create value and should not simply be viewed as a way to delay evaluation and treatment.

ICU FAST TRACKING

Clearly, ICU patients have unique and extreme needs with regard to their care. They are the most critically ill and injured patients we treat, so we need to get it right. But we must also get it as quickly as possible, since many studies have shown that delays in getting patients to the ICU result in worse outcomes. Several healthcare systems, including Intermountain Healthcare in Utah, have established Priority One or ICU Fast Track programs to put order sets and protocols guided by EBM in place for ICU patients.

When patients with identified diagnoses present to the ED, such as those in the list below, a team is activated that includes, at a minimum, an ICU nurse and an intensivist or a mid-level provider, who come to the ED or inpatient unit within a specified time frame (usually 30 minutes or less) and evaluate the patient for an expedited transfer to the ICU.

ICU Fast Tracking Criteria

Those diagnoses and symptoms warranting ICU Fast Tracking include the following:

- Sepsis or sepsis syndrome
- Resuscitation post–cardiac arrest
- Acute respiratory failure requiring mechanical ventilation
- Unstable hemodynamics requiring vasopressor support
- Intracranial hemorrhage with evolving neurologic signs and/or airway compromise
- Monitoring requirements including arterial line, pulmonary wedge catheters, and intracranial pressure monitors

In our experience, the Priority One and ICU Fast Track programs have resulted in dramatic reductions in time to ICU from 300 minutes to less than 60 minutes.

EVIDENCE-BASED ADMITTING CRITERIA

Evidence-based admitting criteria are a set of demand–capacity management principles adapted to the inpatient side of the ledger. They contain clearly understood orders for the most commonly admitted patient types on the inpatient service, including diagnostic and therapeutic elements. Emergency physicians and hospitalists are then on the same page because they are looking at the same set of clinical orders, whose establishment was guided by Centers for Medicare & Medicaid Services (CMS) Core Measures and generally accepted EBM.

We have to use the tools of demand–capacity management to predict how the most common admissions will be evaluated and treated, develop EBM protocols to address them, and hold the team accountable for both compliance and results. Evidence from the implementation of these programs has shown a dramatic improvement in length of stay, CMS Core Measure compliance, and patient and staff satisfaction (Mayer and Jensen 2013). We believe this is one of the most productive areas of inpatient flow and produces a dramatic return on investment for those hospitals and healthcare systems that have embraced it as a part of their culture.

All of these—and many other—strategies are at the core of our collective efforts to improve hospitalwide flow.

FLOW AND THE PSYCHOLOGY OF WAITING

Waiting is always difficult. Waiting when your health and safety are potentially in question can be intolerable. In our society, information moves at the speed of electrons. People do not. Systems do not. Yet we expect them to. We need to get used to that reality and figure out how to deal with it in our professional lives. Fortunately, psychologist David Maister (2005) has put a great deal of thought and analysis into this issue. He notes eight core observations in his work "The Psychology of Waiting Lines." While his observations were not specifically in response to healthcare system scenarios, they are definitely applicable to them:

1. Occupied waits are better than unoccupied waits.
2. In-process waits are better than pre-process waits.
3. Anxiety makes waits seem longer.
4. Uncertain waits seem longer than known, finite waits.
5. Unexplained waits are longer than explained waits.

6. Unfair waits are longer than equitable waits.
7. The more valuable the service, the longer the wait is tolerable.
8. Solo waits feel longer than group waits.

Let's take a quick look at how each of these concepts can be put to work to deal with the waiting—which, unfortunately, often is an ingrained part of the delivery of healthcare, despite our best efforts to improve flow by adding value and eliminating waste (particularly waiting).

Occupied waits are better than unoccupied waits and can be facilitated by providing these items:

- Magazines
- Healthcare informational material
- Interactive video healthcare messages
- Healthcare kiosks
- E-mail or Internet access
- TVs, iPods, and other media formats

In-process waits are better than pre-process waits and can be enhanced by using the following processes:

- Direct-to-bed and triage bypass
- Team triage
- Getting the doctor and patient together as soon as possible
- Front-loading flow

Anxiety makes waits seem longer but can be decreased by these methods:

- Making the customer service diagnosis
- Addressing the patient's problem rapidly
- Getting information to the patient as quickly as possible
- Using scripts to reduce anxiety; for example, "This doesn't look like a heart attack and your EKG is normal, but let's get some blood work and monitor your heart rhythm to be sure."

Uncertain waits seem longer than known, finite waits but can be eased by the following strategies:

- Giving previews—letting the patient and family know what is going to happen
- Expectation creation
- Sharing dashboards that show expected wait times in the following manner:
  - Green (open, quick service)
  - Yellow (some delays expected)
  - Red (delays near certain)
- Providing test and consult results as soon as possible

Unexplained waits are longer than explained waits but can be eased by

- explaining to patients who are waiting when high-acuity events occur, such as trauma, code strokes, cardiac arrests, or operating room delays for unstable patients;
- keeping patients and their families posted on the progress of tests, transfers, and discharges; and
- providing accurate estimates of consults, services, and diagnostic evaluations.

Unfair waits are longer than equitable waits but can be eased by these tactics:

- Explaining services such as Fast Track, outpatient elective versus major surgery, and staged surgery
- Leading up on delays and the reasons for them
- Using occupied time (see earlier bullet point) to make the delays seem shorter

The *more valuable the service*, the longer the wait is tolerable when you and your staff

- accentuate benefits and eliminate burdens,
- communicate this concept through the use of scripts, and
- provide ongoing assessment of patient and family expectations.

Solo waits feel longer than group waits but can be improved by

- having liberal family visitation policies;
- occupying any known downtime when the patient will be alone, for example, with child-life programs in pediatrics or the use of social work and case management; and
- offering family conference updates.

Maister's insights have many, many applications. Put your team to work to tap their creative empowerment to discover ways in which they can apply these observations for the good of the patient and share the insights across the organization.

FLOW AS THE FINAL FRONTIER?

In some ways, flow is like the final frontier (you know, from *Star Trek*?) in that flow addresses the entire patient experience, not just the perception patients have of the service we provide. As we've mentioned before, the advent of the HCAHPS survey, which is much more of a patient experience survey than simply a service survey, accentuates the importance of having not just A-Team members but also A-Team processes, designed and driven by the evidence collected throughout the care of the patient and fed back to the providers of that care so they can further and continuously refine how that care is provided. And in our current capacity-constrained environments, where we are challenged to be the high-quality, low-cost providers of care by doing more with less (IHI 2005), flow is an essential tool to drive the successful implementation of healthcare processes and services.

SURVIVAL SKILLS SUMMARY

- *Flow* is defined as the ability to add value and eliminate waste as our patients move through the service transitions and queues that healthcare comprises.
- Value is defined as a ratio of the benefits received divided by the burdens endured in the course of the delivery of that care.
- Leaders must be on a treasure hunt to identify and accentuate value and a bounty hunt to identify and eliminate waste on behalf of the patient.
- Over time, A-Team members can be beaten down by the incessant demands of B-Team processes.
- Implementing the principles of flow has an importance to the legitimate assessment of our leadership. Are we up to the challenge of increasing value and eliminating waste?
- There are many examples of ED and healthcare-wide flow—how many more will you and your team add?
- Use the psychology of waiting to put your team to work to find ways to make delays more tolerable.

REFERENCES

Berwick, D. M., and A. D. Hackbarth. 2012. "Eliminating Waste in US Healthcare." *Journal of the American Medical Association* 307 (14): 362.

Institute for Healthcare Improvement (IHI). 2005. *Going Lean in Health Care.* IHI Innovation Series white paper. www.ihi.org/resources/Pages/IHIWhitePapers/GoingLeaninHealthCare.aspx.

Jensen, K., T. A. Mayer, S. J. Welch, and C. Haraden. 2007. *Leadership for Smooth Patient Flow: Improved Outcomes, Improved Service, Improved Bottom Line.* Chicago: Health Administration Press.

Maister, D. H. 2005. "The Psychology of Waiting Lines." http://davidmaister.com/wp-content/themes/davidmaister/pdf/PsycholgyofWaitingLines751.pdf.

Mayer, T. 2005. "Team Triage and Treatment, Be a Bed Ahead, and Adopt a Boarder." Accessed October 7, 2013. http://smhs.gwu.edu/urgentmatters/sites/urgentmatters/files/enewslettcr_volume2_issue1_TeamTriage_Mayer.pdf.

Mayer, T., and K. Jensen. 2013. "Hardwiring Hospital-wide and ED Flow." Seminar presented to the American College of Healthcare Executives Congress on Healthcare Leadership, Chicago, March 12.

———. 2012. "The Business Case for Patient Flow." *Healthcare Executive* 27 (4): 50–53.

———. 2009. *Hardwiring Flow: Systems and Processes for Seamless Patient Care.* Gulf Breeze, FL: Fire Starter Press.

Porter, M. E. 2010. "What Is Value in Health Care?" *New England Journal of Medicine* 363 (26): 2477–81.

Porter, M. E., and T. L. Lee. 2013. "The Strategy That Will Fix Healthcare." *Harvard Business Review* 91 (10): 51–70.

Toussaint, J. S., and L. L. Berry. 2013. "The Promise of Lean in Health Care." *Mayo Clinic Proceedings* 88 (1): 74–82.

CHAPTER 16

A-Team Tool 9—Rewarding Champions

The concept of rewarding your champions is simply to recognize the legitimate role praise plays in continuously motivating professionals. One of the best ways to ensure that your staff members feel like heroes is to tell them—and tell them, and tell them. You cannot praise them enough.

You can take a systematic, visible, and meaningful approach to celebrating the successes visibly and meaningfully. The following steps are suggestions for institutionalizing a program of rewarding the champions at your organization.

1. Use your metrics-based reports to identify accomplishments. Flow metrics, service scores, Core Measures compliance, bed turns, and other measures that are routinely kept track of allow us to notice when things are working well in our hospitals. Many of us can even see these metrics from the computer screens in our offices. Take the time to reach out to those leaders and managers whose metrics support their championship-caliber efforts.

2. Share the stories of your "service legends." Celebrate the successes of your service champions by sharing service legend stories at every management or leadership team meeting. Read letters from patients complimenting staff; better yet, ask the patients to attend the meeting, tell their story, and present the service award. Every meeting should feature at least one such commendation and, in our opinion, should have this activity at the top of the agenda.

3. Send personal notes as a follow-up to patients' letters. When you receive copies of the compliment letters sent by patients, send a personal note of recognition (handwritten whenever possible) to the staff members identified in the letters, as in the following example:

Betsy,

I had a chance to see the wonderful note from Mrs. Smith—a great example of your A-Team attitude. Thanks so much for your help in making our hospital the nation's service excellence leader!

Many thanks,

Patrick
CEO
Central Medical Center

4. Post the letters from patients in the staff lounge. Don't just file the letters away. Place them prominently in staff gathering areas so others can help celebrate the success as well as learn from the A-Team behaviors that generated the letters.

5. Institute a "caught caring" program. Find ways to let patients and other staff help celebrate the service excellence they see. At Inova Health System, we have used the "caught caring" approach, whereby we make Post-it-style notes readily available throughout the organization so patients and staff can express their appreciation on the spot. We encourage you to have fun in designing these notes, as Inova has done (see Exhibit 16.1). Inova uses a star theme as part of our champion-rewarding documents, as further illustrated in step 6.

Exhibit 16.1: "Caught Caring" Notes

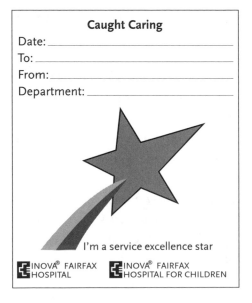

Source: Inova Health System. Used with permission.

---

6. Create a "Star in the ER" program. In our emergency department, we created the Star (as in *starfish*) of the ER award, a visible and meaningful way to reward our champions. Each month, the employee with the best customer service ratings is given the Star of the ER award, which includes a plaque with his or her name and the starfish symbol on it and gift certificates totaling $200. Every three months, a Star of the Quarter is named, who receives a MasterCard gift card worth $500; suite tickets to a local professional hockey, football, or basketball game (depending on the season); and two free first-class airline tickets (donated from the hundreds of thousands of miles we travel each year teaching customer service courses).

The form we use to take nominations for Star of the ER and Star of the Quarter is shown in Exhibit 16.2. It incorporates the concepts of the star and the heart to convey the essence of customer service.

Does this award program cost money? Of course. Does it pay dividends in terms of employee satisfaction? You bet. It is a very small price to pay for letting our staff know how deeply they are appreciated.

7. Use the accolades as leverage to move from 4s to 5s in customer service. Follow the letters, e-mails, and phone calls of praise and use them to help raise the bar for the entire staff. Analyzing A-Team and B-Team behaviors is essential in creating a culture of service. (While A-Team behaviors should be dealt with publicly and with liberal praise, reprimands of B-Team behaviors should always be handled privately, yet expeditiously.)

8. Handle the B-Team issues. By far the best way to reward your champions is to deal with B-Team members and B-Team behaviors. The best gift you can give your high performers is a work environment where they can consistently expect to work with A-Team members.

Exhibit 16.2: H.E.A.R.T./S.T.A.R. Nomination Form

H.E.A.R.T./S.T.A.R

- ❤ Hear the complaint
- ❤ Empathize and evaluate
- ❤ Apolgize
- ❤ Resolve with urgency
- ❤ Thank the patient/
  family member

- ☆ Service
- ☆ Teamwork
- ☆ Accountability
- ☆ Respect

Person nominated:_____

Core Behavior Exhibited:_____

☐ Hear the complaint ☐ Empathize ☐ Apologize ☐ Resolve with urgency ☐ Thank You
☐ Service ☐ Teamwork ☐ Accountability ☐ Respect

Source: Department of Emergency Medicine, Inova Fairfax Hospital. Used with permission.

BENEFITS OF REWARDING YOUR CHAMPIONS

In financial terms, rewarding your champions has the best return on investment of any program in your healthcare system. These initiatives improve employee satisfaction, create service excellence legends, engender excitement about the work, and increase staff retention.

SURVIVAL SKILLS SUMMARY

- A program of rewarding your champions recognizes the role that immediate feedback and praise can play in motivating professionals and team members in that it appeals to their inner desire for excellence.
- Use the data-driven metrics built into your system to prospectively identify high performers and reward them.
- Make service legend stories a routine part of management team meetings. Put it first on the agenda.
- Use handwritten notes to compliment staff. People save notes—they rarely save e-mails.
- Post complimentary letters and e-mails in the staff lounge.
- Find ways to make it easy for patients to compliment staff and for staff to compliment each other, such as through a "caught caring" program.
- Create monthly, quarterly, and yearly service "Star" awards (subject, of course, to the organization's guidelines).
- Praise liberally and publicly. Counsel the B-Team privately.
- Trend A-Team and B-Team compliments/complaints.
- By far most important, the best way to reward your champions is to hold B-Team members accountable. Give the A-Team a work environment where they can expect excellence—from themselves and the entire team.

MORE RESOURCES ON REWARDING CHAMPIONS

Mayer, T. 2010. "Drive Service Excellence to the Next Level." *Healthcare Executive* 25 (6): 54–56.

Peters, T. 2010. *The Little Big Things: 163 Ways to Pursue Excellence.* New York: HarperBusiness.

CHAPTER 17

A-Team Tool 10—Leaving a Legacy

Who among us doesn't want to leave a legacy? Given the incredible difficulty of delivering excellence in both the clinical and service realms, why would anyone ever even remotely consider doing this terribly tough job unless he or she had the innate sense that all this labor, trouble, and concern was somehow *worth* it?

And *how* do we define the worth of what we do in service to our patients? We've talked about adding value and eliminating waste, the benefit/burden ratio, and many other ways of quantifying the value-added concepts of healthcare. All of that is valid and relevant. But are those strategies all we need to motivate others—and ourselves? We all agree that becoming the high-quality, low-cost provider of care and creating value and eliminating waste are necessary conditions—they *must* be there to ensure success in our increasingly capacity-constrained and competitive environment. But are they *sufficient* conditions—do they constitute and create the conditions for success? Again, to quote Nietzsche, "He who has a strong enough 'Why' can bear almost any 'How.'"

Why do those of us in healthcare do this incredibly tough work? It is really very simple, but we need to take a moment to make the "why" a bit more clear. As we've noted before, *all language has meaning, and all behavior has meaning.* What do the language and behavior of our daily lives in healthcare mean? My (TM) son Kevin was asking for help with his homework when he was about 12 years old. Kevin is now a brave and decorated Marine veteran with two tours embedded with Afghan Special Forces in the most perilous of deployments, but back then he asked for help with his homework. I, naively, answered, "Kevin, this is what it *says*," pointing to the instructions from the teacher. Kevin replied, with the wisdom of the child, "Dad, I know what it *says*. But what does it *mean*?"

So what does it mean to leave a legacy? Dictionary definitions do not do the word justice, as they focus on modern, inadequate phrases such as, "something (such as property or money) that is received from someone who has died" (Merriam-Webster 2013). But a more careful look into the origins of the word tells an entirely different story; the etymology of the word *legacy* is fascinating and enlightening. The ancient French derivations of the word refer to "something handed down" and a "body of persons sent on a mission." Medieval Latin roots refer to "an ambassador or envoy sent on a special mission" (Barnhart 1988).

This approximates what we mean by a legacy. We are not referring to the amount of money or property left to our family. As important and admirable as that calculus is, it is not remotely what we are talking about when we say "leave a legacy." We are all ambassadors, individuals on a mission for the benefit of our patients, in the hope of handing down something of value in our service to them. In healthcare we have the most honorable and privileged position imaginable, because we have a unit of measure for our legacy that we can—and most definitely should—measure each and every day. Its measure is not fiscal, strategic, tactical, or even goal oriented. But its measure cannot be avoided, in either its drama or its importance. What is the measure of our legacy? It is simply and eternally this:

In healthcare, our legacy is measured by the simplest and yet most stark of metrics— one patient at a time. Each patient we care for is our legacy.

Where else can anyone finish his day, walk to his car, and ask the question, "What was my legacy *today*?" and be able to answer, "I made a *difference* in the lives of my patients and their families." One patient at a time, one family at a time, we do our best. Is it enough? That is a judgment necessarily left to others. It is not our job or our calling to judge if we have done enough. But have we done the best *we* can do?

Encourage your team members—each day, every day—to take that moment when they sit in their car after a busy, taxing, emotionally draining day/evening/ night shift to ask, "What sort of legacy did I *leave* in there today?"

As we said in the "star thrower" story in Chapter 6, the answer should always be, "I'm a *hero*. I make a difference in the lives of others!" Your team should know that—you should constantly tell them that they are heroes. They need to be reminded of that, and so do you. We are called to a great and noble profession—to serve others with all of our might and soul and sinew. But what a wonderful job it is—and will always be.

Our great friend and mentor Chuck Stokes, FACHE, brought to our attention the following example that illustrates leaving a legacy. The great scientist and philosopher George Washington Carver stated:

How far you go in life depends upon . . .

Before we share the rest of the quote, take a moment to finish that statement for yourself. Perhaps even take the time to write down how you would finish it. Ask your team to do the same. How would they finish "How far you go in life depends upon . . ."?

Now, consider how George Washington Carver finished that statement:

How far you go in life depends upon your being tender with the young, compassionate with the aged, sympathetic to the striving and tolerant of the weak and strong. Because someday in your life, you will have been *all* of those things.

This philosophy constantly resonates within us. *Every day*, we have the great privilege, by necessity, of continuously being

- *tender with the young,*
- *compassionate with the aged,*
- *sympathetic with the striving, and*
- *tolerant of the weak and strong, because*
- *every day you will serve all of these people.*

To be called to the great and noble work in which we not only can leave a legacy every day we work but also can measure that legacy, one patient at a time:

What a challenge.
What a responsibility.
What a burden.
And, ultimately, what a joy.

What better legacy can we in healthcare leave?

REFERENCES

Barnhart, R. E. (ed.). 1988. *Barnhart's Dictionary of Etymology*. New York: H.W. Wilson.

Merriam-Webster Online. 2013. "Legacy." www.merriam-webster.com/dictionary/legacy.

About the Authors

Thom A. Mayer, MD, is founder and chief executive officer of BestPractices, Inc., and an executive vice president of EmCare, the nation's largest provider of emergency physician services and a national resource in physician leadership and management. He also serves as the medical director for the NFL Players Association and for the Studer Group.

Dr. Mayer has been the keynote speaker at numerous healthcare leadership conferences. He was named the American College of Emergency Physicians (ACEP) Outstanding Speaker of the Year in the second year the award was given and has won the Over the Top award from ACEP, which recognizes the organization's highest-rated speaker, a record five times. He is a featured speaker at the American College of Healthcare Executives' (ACHE) Senior Executive and Executive programs. He is one of America's foremost experts on healthcare customer service, trauma and emergency care, pediatric emergency care, and medical leadership. He has published more than 100 articles and 120 book chapters and has edited 20 medical textbooks. Dr. Mayer is coeditor with Robert W. Strauss of *Strauss and Mayer's Emergency Department Management*, considered by many to be the benchmark text on emergency leadership. His book with Kirk Jensen, Shari J. Welch, and Carol Haraden, *Leadership for Smooth Patient Flow: Improved Outcomes, Improved Service, Improved Bottom Line,* was the winner of ACHE's 2008 James A. Hamilton Award for healthcare management book of the year.

On September 11, 2001, Dr. Mayer served as one of the command physicians at the Pentagon Rescue Operation, coordinating medical assets at the site. The BestPractices physicians at Inova Fairfax Hospital were the first to successfully diagnose and treat inhalational anthrax victims during the 2001 anthrax crises. Dr. Mayer has also served the US Department of Defense on the Defense Science Board's Task Forces on Bioterrorism, Weapons of Mass Destruction, and Homeland Security.

Robert J. (Bob) Cates, MD, is a practicing emergency department physician and chairman of Inova Fairfax Hospital's Department of Emergency Medicine in Falls Church, Virginia. Under Dr. Cates's leadership, the emergency department has won numerous awards and grants, most recently the prestigious Robert Wood Johnson Foundation Urgent Matters Grant. One of the ten busiest emergency departments in the country, it nonetheless sustains the highest levels of patient satisfaction. It is widely recognized for providing innovative and cutting-edge solutions for patient flow and service.

Dr. Cates received his undergraduate degree at Southern Illinois University, his master's degree in biochemistry at Indiana University, and his MD degree at Indiana University. His postgraduate training included a medicine internship at Indiana University Medical Center, a medicine residency at Georgetown University, and four years as a clinical associate and staff associate at the National Institutes of Health in the National Cancer Institute. He is a widely sought-after speaker on the application of customer service in healthcare.